JOURNEY INWARD

JOURNEY INWARD

A Walk Toward Victory Over the Ego

NARDU DEBRAH

Foreword by John Danaher

Copyright © 2020

All rights reserved

First paperback edition June 2020

Interior design by Lexy Alemao

1 3 5 7 9 10 8 6 4 2

ISBN 978-0-578-68507-6

www.journeyinward.site

*Dedicated to my family, friends, students,
and all my martial arts teachers who were gracious enough
to impart their knowledge and wisdom to me,
especially my Sifu Ralph Mitchell.*

Three Blessings

To give a man a sword.

To teach him precisely how to maintain and wield the sword.

To teach him precisely when and when not to use the sword.

Table of Contents

Foreword   xi
Preface   1
Introduction   3

1: Get Punched in the Face   7

2: Get Tapped Out   13

3: Courtesy the Mat   19

4: Take Ukemi/Be a Uke   25

5: Fold Your Gi   35

6: Step into the Ring   41

7: Clean the Blade   49

8: See the End Result and Be Nothing   57

Table of Contents

9: Go Through the Dark Side   63

10: Give Back   71

Instructions on Awakening   *79*
Closing   *81*
About the Author   *83*
Glossary   *85*
Photos   *91*

Foreword

The last three decades have seen an enormous change in martial arts. This revolution was started by the rise of mixed martial arts competition. The age-old question of which martial arts style was the most effective was put to the test in the cauldron of the mixed martials arts cage. For a time, each style seemed to have risen to prominence, only to be eclipsed by some new style that, in turn, was eclipsed by another until the answer became clear: They all work well if applied well and in integration with the others.

A side effect of this revolution was an effective split of the martial arts into traditional schools, which tended to emphasize a single approach to combat along with character development; and modern schools, which tended to emphasize integrated approaches to combat and physical development. This split was understandable but unfortunate, as both approaches have much to offer the other.

Nardu Debrah is one of the rare martial artists today with a lifelong commitment to both schools of thought. He has integrated them successfully into his life and the lives of his many students.

He began in traditional martial arts in New York City. When the mixed martial arts revolution began, he competed very successfully as a mixed martial arts athlete during the early growth of the sport here in the United States. He then went on to coach it at the highest levels, with standout UFC athletes under his guidance. He has lived both lives at the highest levels.

I have watched him grow as an athlete and coach over two decades. Even to this day he seeks out the latest innovations and evolutions to stay current in a turbulent and rapidly changing sport. What sets him apart, however, is that in the midst of all this change and turmoil, he is grounded in the ways of the traditional arts. His approach is always that the mind is the governor of the body and that cultivation of our mental outlook is the basis of a lifelong commitment to improvement in a physical art.

By reconciling traditional and modern approaches to the combat arts and sports, he espouses a view that makes martial arts more than a way of attaining physical ascendency over others and makes it about ascension over ourselves—for only when this is achieved can we pursue martial arts not for a championship or a belt, but for a lifetime of improvement of ourselves and those around us.

Watching the growth of Nardu Debrah has been a pleasure over the many years I have known him. Seeing him take the deep lessons he has learned and taught to his students here in New York to a wider audience with this work only adds to that pleasure.

—John Danaher

JOURNEY INWARD

Preface

Any and all writings in this book are solely of my origin.

If there is any error, it is of my own and not of the great masters before me. I will give you, in my most sincere account, the methods you need to improve your life and the world. These methods are not easy and are painstaking.

Yet, in the end, when you see the grand ocean view, you will know that you have in this lifetime become free of trappings, yearnings, and attachments, and you have rid yourself of all sickness of the mind. You have gained victory over the ego. With clarity, you will smile at the dawn of luminosity. You will know that no stone has been left unturned, and that true freedom can be attained.

These may just be the grumblings of an unshaven martial artist. However, I will assure you that if you begin on your journey today, it will be a good day for you and the world.

Let us see the natural simplicity of what will be said here. That is, if we want to improve society, we must start with ourselves. To improve ourselves, we must shine a light on our weak areas. Then, we must go inward to find the cause of our ignorance. There is where our ego sits. Once the ego is found, we still have to go deeper and begin to extract, dissolve, or put to use.

All that is without, first comes from within. To go inward, it will take courage. To sit alone with yourself in silence will speak volumes to who you are. Courage will be necessary, and I am certain that you can do it. You may have to walk through some difficult doors, but inward fortitude is a must. It is said that to have knowledge and not contribute is to share the road of the greedy, so I have decided to put to paper some teachings from my experience that will help you on your path. But do not confuse knowledge with knowing.

This is not a course for linear logic. It is for you to observe inwardly and see the truth of yourself. Ego can be defined as a person's self-esteem or self-worth. We cannot put an end to the ego. As long as we have breath, our ego will breathe with us. My intention is not to capture and detain the ego. That would not be possible, as the ego is intangible. What we will set out to do is observe. Observe inwardly our thoughts and emotions. I want to give you a tool that is of great importance in any endeavor, especially in a self-defense situation. That tool is called awareness. Make no mistake, this is indeed self-defense.

The capacity to gain an accurate and deep, intuitive understanding of a person or thing is what defines insight. It is to see the spirit of a thing for what it is and not what it appears to be. Together, with awareness as your guide and insight as your light, you now have the necessary tools to help you navigate inwardly. You have now entered into the correct view. You are now ready to embark on your journey. Travel well.

Introduction

It is my stance of no stance that martial arts and the Budo tradition nourish the mind, body, and soul. Just as food and water give our physical body vitality, so too does the study of Budo nurture us. This book is for those looking to improve their life by learning how to go within, examine the ego, and merge with the infinite potential of the correct view. You, the reader, will have to take action, perform a self-examination. It will be difficult. However, in the end you will know how to keep your center and not get taken off balance—physically and mentally.

It is my stance of no stance that a person must embark on the journey of learning the martial arts, in some way, either at a school or from another individual. The learning of the arts is a necessity for thoroughly understanding the writings and lessons in this book.

It is my stance of no stance that you, the reader, must meditate on these words. The reader must know that these words are just the gate. They are not the house, and you must go through the gate to reach the house. Seeing this, you must remember that the teacher often points the direction. However, it is you who must walk down the path.

It is my stance of no stance that Budo principles and the study of the martial arts can heal an individual, thus society, thus a nation, and, ultimately, the world. The source of most healing is looked for outside of oneself—to a deity or an absolute truth beyond the mind. The keys have been in your hand all along. But it takes tremendous courage, not to journey outward, but to journey inward.

To begin to see the truth of it all is the important thing—to see something for what it is and not what it appears to be. To have an insight into it. As I write this book, there is a global pandemic going on. A virus has attacked mankind. There is death and sorrow everywhere. Due to the nature of this particular virus, human beings have been forced to be separated, to isolate and keep a certain distance as much as possible.

This will be done temporarily to curb the spread of this virus. It is as though nature is telling mankind that it is time to put away our outer illusions and go within. We often build up an identity and begin hoarding things toward that identity. We even build fences to say, "This is mine." We produce brands, labels, and other illusions.

Then, nature sends a great wave. The force of this wave smashes away all in its path, including you. Then, once the tide settles, there will be little left. The virus facing mankind does not discriminate. Although we have our own sacred spaces, nature has been trying to remind us that we are not separate from it. When the wind blows, we all feel it. When it rains, we all get wet, and when a virus invades, we all take cover.

Yet, there is still the mischievous one, the ego within us. The man whose ego is unchecked loses humility. The loss of humility disconnects him from the ground. He begins to float away. He believes he is better, more refined, more civil, more intelligent than the rest. His castle is better, has deeper moats and more fortified towers. He holds his chin higher and proclaims himself as the emperor.

Then nature comes along and sends a great earthquake. The castle has come to ruin. Yet inwardly, all that built the castle remains intact, including the ego. We are not separate from nature, and we are not separate from the ego.

The key is to put everything in its right place, to see that we are all interconnected. Many talk of karma yet fail to go further and study Dharma, which is simply the inherent nature of reality, or a universal truth. It is important not to just skim the surface but to go deeper, to journey inward to find the healing. Natural disasters are often nature's way of humbling mankind, as he continually takes and hurts nature for his own gains.

I have shared a few of my experiences on my journey in the martial arts, experiences that brought me to the greater truth that martial arts point us to—that is, improving or mastering the self, helping others to master themselves; lighting your inner light, then helping others kindle theirs. If light can be found within, ignorance gets expelled without. But it will not be easy. I will share with you some steps on my path. However, ultimately you will have to walk a path of your own.

If I could impart a few insights to you, then the seed will be planted. Tatsuya Nakadai told me that sometimes we plant stones and sometimes we plant seeds. However, sometimes we think we planted a stone, yet later it turns out to be a seed. This is because of the judgment of nature. So time and experience is a critical thing. Time gives us experience and teaches us wisdom. The important thing is not to rush. Do not stop and start. Once you begin training, you must be consistent. In terms of the martial arts, you must learn the art in its entirety, not in fragments.

I have laid out what needs to be done. However, do not take a quick fix approach or seek instant enlightenment. Instead, I want you to just walk, one step at a time, closer and closer to yourself, inward to where the ego rests. Find a quiet place. Take your time when you read this book, more understanding will come as you mature. Together we will free the ego of all its grasping, yearning, and attachments. We will, in essence, cleanse the vision so we can see the spirit of a thing, improve ourselves, and improve the world.

www.journeyinward.site

1
Get Punched in the Face

*"If you are not a humble person,
fighting will bring humbleness to you."*
—Mike Tyson—

It is of the utmost importance that you, yes you, get punched in the face. Preferably with a boxing glove, 12 or 16 ounces will do. But I mean a real punch, not a love tap, light jab, or a pitty-pat touch. When you get hit, you will be forced to journey inward. You will immediately have to ask yourself a few simple questions: "Do I want to continue?" "What just happened?" "Could I take another shot?" "How did I get caught?" "Where was my opening?" "Where was my defense?"

If you were hit so hard that you went unconscious, then do not worry about all the above, because you will feel only the after effects of a hangover and will not remember much of what occurred. However, the residual pain will be a reminder that you have been touched in a particular, pugilistic way.

Whether you were a humble person to begin with or the opposite, getting hit is the best thing for your soul. While this is not something that should keep occurring, it is something that should happen from time to time and at different levels, depending on your experience or lack thereof.

So, what is the magic in getting hit? It keeps you grounded. Naturally, it gives you clarity. There is only one thing we know about generals who are ready to die: That is, they can be killed. First, you must realize that you can be hit. You have openings, flaws, and imperfections in your defense—areas in your movement and choices that you must improve.

For a beginner, there is often a feeling of embarrassment, especially if others are watching. For the advanced, there is also a feeling of embarrassment, but its seed lies in a remarkable place, a place we are approaching in great detail and study, a place we call the EGO. I am not talking about a schoolyard scrap or a wild, crazy mess that goes back and forth with unskilled strikes. I am talking about a real punch from someone who understands body mechanics, timing, depth perception, speed, power, and all the rest.

My earliest memory of a real punch in the face was during my teenage years when entering the martial arts school called Universal Defense System under the strict tutelage of Sifu Ralph Mitchell. After every class would be full contact sparring. It was one of the best parts of training. Sparring was where we got to put function to form and where Sifu did not tolerate excuses. So you had to keep it real with yourself and your sparring partner.

Let us briefly talk about the impact, or negative feedback, of the punch and what you will experience.

For a fraction of a second, your eyes will close. Therefore, you will see darkness. The punch will shake your senses, so you may also see bright lights. You will smell the odor of the leather, there will be a feeling of an implosion and explosion simultaneously.

After the hit, your spirit will come to the surface. Fueled by the ego, your next actions are the gap for the ultimate truth of yourself. It is a special place where the ego will reveal itself. Beat the grass to startle the snakes.

Do you have a feeling in the pit of your gut that says, "I gotta get that back," or do you have a sense that says, "Time out, this is not for me"? Either feeling is acceptable because it is called the beginning. At least you were brave enough to take the first step. You actually got punched in the face. You put on gloves, put Vaseline on your face, stood in front of a skilled opponent, and got hit. There is no shame in that. However, your next steps will bring about either great shame or great honor.

Gather yourself. Then enter. That means picking up the pieces. Make your mind anew, then move forward. Both the beginner and the advanced must dissolve this feeling of embarrassment and use it as fuel. It will not be easy, but it must be done. Let us put the ego to good use here. We should work with the ego to allow it to point in two directions, the past and the future, realizing that the punch was your gift—the present. It was a gift that will lead you toward future improvement—to see the strike clearly so that you can defend and improve timing. It was a gift that will point you to the past, to remember the pain, not to go into denial, and not to make excuses.

This goes the same for body shots: a penetrating kick delivered to the abdomen, collapsing the diaphragm; a well-placed right hook that fractures ribs; or, of course, the ultimate liver shot, which can send you down to a knee or balled up on your back in pain.

The body shot has a special feeling. Since you are entirely conscious and your head or eyes have not been touched as bad, you get to be awake and alert the entire time. There is an inner reverberation of pain that blasts into your soul.

It is as if you are shouting with full intensity while completely submerged. A well-placed, well-timed body shot will in fact change your life. If you are sturdy, you can withstand the pain. However, the eyes will change even though the intensity will lessen.

I can recall the thick, heavy smell of Thai liniments, muscle balms, cigarettes, and beer. This is what our changing rooms and warm-up area reeked of. While we stretched and prepared backstage to come to the arena to fight, we never actually had a chance to see the fights happening in the arena. At that time, there were no TVs in the changing area, and promoters did not want to pay any more than they had to for something not necessary.

So backstage, the sense that we used the most was our hearing. There would suddenly be a loud roar. Then a sudden cheer. There would be loud applause for approvals and boos for disapprovals. To us fighters backstage, the event literally sounded like a roller coaster.

The returning fighters came back like modern-day gladiators, soaked in blood and sweat, and their team had the energy of either a wedding or a funeral. Once we were called to the ring, it was as if time was suspended. It was as if we had slipped into a gap, a special place beyond excited, beyond the physical realm.

For a moment, it is as if you are looking at yourself. You begin a systems-ready check. You reflect upon all your blood, sweat, and sacrifice that brought you to the moment. Hours upon hours of grueling training and intense practice stand behind you.

Then, you see it all, all that you have done, and, if you did your homework, you are only one word: ready. The next thing I saw on that day was the center referee looking at me saying, "Are you ready?" My response was, "Hell yeah."

The fight itself is so much simpler than the pre-fight rituals because your mind, body, and spirit are like an arrow with a high-carbon, extremely sharp steel tip. The waiting time is you sitting in the bow being pulled back, ready to be launched.

The magic of the body shot is that you really remember the lessons. Therefore, you know what it can do to another person. In this particular match I was in, it was a mixed martial arts (MMA) bout. So we wore only four-ounce gloves. For me, this was a thing of beauty. I knew that most fighters trained in arts in which the hand was protected while training. So this brought me to exciting territory. In the traditional arts that most MMA fighters do not train in, there is an area of skin, tendon, bone, and marrow conditioning whose sole purpose is to callus the external layer of skin, in particular the hand, knuckle, and forearm.

Due to my many days of three-star blocking and iron shirt drills with Sifu, I already had been through a level of conditioning training that I could only describe as Spartan. So to now have the freedom to hit at will with no rules (or limited rules) was a beautiful thing. During the first round, I landed a body shot on my opponent.

Before that body shot, he was coming at me like hell on wheels. But after the hit landed, there was a sudden halt, a change in his spirit. I saw a look in his eyes as if he were falling into a pit of despair. The energy to advance was utterly taken out of him; it was if his desire to win had completely abandoned him and his will to fight had been checkmated.

In training, your practice must be real. It is a danger to engage in false practice or not give the truth to your training partner. It is in training where the wisdom becomes manifest. The cobwebs clear, the dust and pain settle, and you return to your senses. As you sit there, staring into the moment, you approach the horizon, the inward horizon of your perception.

Sifu Ralph Mitchell would always shout, "Keep your focus!" In other words, regroup, refocus, and get your head back in the game. Do not allow your lower self to pull you into the depths of denial. Put your chin down, keep your hands up, bite down on your mouthpiece, accept the hit, and prepare for more to come as you are learning. You are not losing. Get the correct view. Make sturdy your mind and continue to push forward. Even a trained person's ego can get humbled during a fight. So, the important thing about getting hit is to experience it, then let the lessons seep into your soul.

A good punch in the face will pull you down from your high horse. It is a great starting ground. A good first step on your journey inward.

This understanding is for those who intend to be warriors.

2

Get Tapped Out

*"Our fears don't stop death,
they stop life."*
—Rickson Gracie—

According to the waza, there are only two paths that lead to a submission or getting tapped out. These are a joint lock (kansetsu waza) or strangulation (shime waza). There are, of course, a myriad of methods of deploying these waza, which make the art of Jiujitsu a beautiful, never-ending study. Each of these waza (techniques) carries its own unique beauty, its own level of a finite truth—a definite halt in your opponent's offense, a stop in his will, a finish of a time, a surrender, and an agreement. We call this conclusion a "tap out."

After your relentless struggle to gain a victory, when two warriors begin to engage in newaza, or live grappling, one person will get caught in either a strangulation technique or a joint lock from which they will be forced to tap. It is in this tap where the magic occurs.

Yes, I know it may have been painful. I know you may have gotten injured. But the injures and pain are reminders, and they come with the territory. That injury can also increase depending on how determined you are NOT to tap.

Now that we see the tap as a conclusion to a short story, what do we learn from that story? To understand, we must go deeper. For the beginner, who enters the training hall with no prior training, it is a beautiful thing. Because he has no expectations, he is very much like a newborn baby entering the world trying to explore the house by crawling here, there, everywhere. This type of beginner with no prior training has an empty cup. Therefore, he is able to taste the tea and all its herbal benefits without any interference.

There is, however, another type of beginner. He is called an "expert." Either he is what my Sifu would call a "legend in his own mind" or, due to his prior training, his ability to learn and absorb wholeheartedly is blocked. At first glance, this type of student may appear to be someone not fit to be in the school or learn the way. On the contrary, this type of steel, if appropriately molded, can become one of the sharpest swords of all.

For this student, who may or may not have had prior training but is a tough guy in his head, his ego is right on the surface. Therefore, it becomes a sink or swim situation much more quickly. Either he taps out, throws a fit, and never returns or he gets humbled that someone half his size almost choked him unconscious or snapped one of his limbs. To avoid severe injury, he was forced to tap, to agree that he has more to learn, to agree that he is a beginner, and to agree that he must humble himself and embrace the art.

There is also the student with prior training who enters already with the correct view. This student has come from another martial art in which his ego was already put in check. He has already taken ukemi, hit the makiwara, tasted his own blood, or been pinned during a contest. This student sees getting tapped out from the correct view, which is simply as a means of learning and improving: trial, error, and correction. This mentality of growth will lead to progression on the mats; gaining more and more experience with every session; making fewer errors; and enjoying the shared training, then reciprocating by helping others who enter to do the same.

It is this very tap that makes you dig deep within the abyss of your soul. For a moment, especially with chokes, it is as if you look death right in the eye. Then you are faced with a choice: to tap, or not to tap and figure a way out of the dilemma.

I recall fighting for the very first Ring of Combat Championship, a Lou Neglia promotion at the Mohegan Sun. My opponent had caught me in the beginning of a triangle choke, what we call a trapped triangle, and then closed it to a full triangle. The triangle choke, or sankaku jime, is one of the most devastating and powerful chokes of Jiujitsu because it utilizes the legs to squeeze the neck and compress the arteries of the neck.

Ultimately, Jiujitsu is a problem-solving or dilemma-solving science, but there is also the spirit of a thing. When I was inside the choke, I can only describe it as a feeling of drowning coupled with the muffled cheers of the arena. However, in that chaotic moment, when there seemed to be no way out, I had to journey inward to a special place beyond the pain, beyond the tap, and beyond the moment. I had summoned every ounce of experience, grit, and determination to ultimately free myself from the choke and go on to win the championship. There is no way I could have journeyed beyond those doors if I had not been tapped out hundreds of times during training. It is the accumulation of taps that brings you towards greatness. It is the accumulated waves crashing into the rocks that give them their beauty, and it is the accumulated hammering of steel that ultimately can forge the finest and sharpest of swords.

I have noticed a sharp contrast between the martial artist who taps and the martial artist who trains in an art where tapping is not a part of the training. The difference is humility. This extends to all people. Grappling arts, such as Jiujitsu, offer us a new paradigm of problem-solving.

It is as though we are arresting a water cat. He is tough to pin down and also very elusive. In order to control or pin this type of cat, working in sectors and closing in space is critical. There will be a particular mind needed to pin this type of opponent.

But there are other opponent types. One is the "silverback gorilla." Due to his powerful nature, it may first appear as if you do not stand a chance. Then there is, of course, the "hawk." He flies and has a speed like no other. To deal with him, you must capture his wings. When you deal with the "octopus" type, you cannot leave too many openings because he will find them and move into them. Meanwhile, the "piranhas" you face have razor-sharp teeth, so working in tight quarters may not be suitable.

It is said that we must respond like an echo and adapt like a shadow. This ability to adapt, to have a solid plan and be prepared to pivot and adjust, comes from being on the mats with all the incredible training partners who will give you various energies.

So, we see getting tapped out is just as important as going for the tap, attempting with every fiber in your being to seize the leopard and make him tap. As the opponent escapes one submission attempt, you throw up another and another, until ultimately you secure position and they tap.

When your opponent taps, there is a new danger that arises. You have had a small success. The small success can go to your head. There is a danger of becoming arrogant. However, the arrogance comes from those who are not on the mats. If you stay on the mats enough, you will also get tapped out or realize there is still more to learn.

So, the important thing is balance. If you are in a state of continually getting submitted and having no moments of small success, it is easy to become demoralized. It is that balance of submitting and getting submitted that keeps the ego in its right place.

We learn that what works for one person may not work for another, and what you envisioned working so perfectly may not have been the best attack of choice. So we learn not to always see in absolutes but to see as a good farmer does—to give the crops space, just like humor gives the mind space. We learn not to be so one-dimensional, but to diversify attack and defense.

So in essence, you are learning to flow and crash, to be silent yet loud, to be swift and slow, light and dark. You are becoming the embodied living principle of yin and yang.

The martial artist who does not tap is lacking. Here, the tap means literally tap. This should not be taken as a metaphor. You need to feel your limbs being taken to the breaking point. You need to feel your arteries losing circulation due to a vice-grip choke. It is there where you will learn to keep your feet on the ground and be humble.

So what if you tap out everyone in the dojo? Maybe you are the highest in rank or instructor. This is the time to move beyond your dojo and travel, meet other warriors on the path. Sometimes simple conversations with other Budoka can hit you with a lifetime of wisdom with just one small chat.

Remember, the writings in this book will free you of yearning, grasping, and attaching. The ego will also be set straight. However, you cannot pick and choose if you have strength and progress in one area, then move to another.

We cannot forget the most crucial aspect that comes along with getting tapped out. That is, it directs us towards the master.

It leads us back to shoshin (beginner's mind). It keeps us in a constant state of evolving, not revolving. We must again sit at the master's feet. Stop, look, listen, and take the next most important step: Ask and humbly receive.

This understanding is for those who intend to be warriors.

3
Courtesy the Mat

*"The final goal of Judo discipline is to perfect yourself
and contribute something to the world."*
—Jigoro Kano—

A man once came to my school and said, "I notice you bow to the mats." I replied, "Yes." He asked, "If I join your dojo, I do not have to bow to the mats, do I? We are not orientals." I simply smiled and directed him to another place that may have fit his needs better.

It was then that I realized more than ever the importance of reiho, or for our purposes, courtesy. The fact that he saw the simple gesture of respect through a cultural lens explains the lack in the world and in mankind.

Reiho is at the heart of an awakened mind, and for one to see its importance, one must journey inward. The landscape of the training hall is important: a clean open space that is devoid of clutter and a safe place to train and grow in. The mindscape, however, is also essential. In the so-called traditional martial arts, there is a great sense of legacy and the passing down of the art from a grandmaster to a master, then to you. You are what we call a keeper of the record. You join a lineage of a rich heritage that, in some cases, has lasted over centuries. That torch has been passed down to you. In a dojo, you will often see pictures of the martial arts ancestry. For example, in many Judo schools there will be a picture of Kano Jigoro Sensei. In BJJ schools, you may see photos of Carlos Gracie or Helio Gracie, etc.

These ancestors are vital, and you must know who they are. They were keepers of the way. It is because of their sacrifice that you can now learn and enjoy that particular martial art. Even though you never met them, as they long ago passed away, you should feel a sense of obligation as a new student to learn, appreciate, and even enhance or transcend their martial art. You are now a keeper of the way, and your picture will possibly one day be on a dojo wall if you aspire to great heights in your training and bring forth the genius inside you.

We must be clear that when we bow or courtesy to the ancestors, we are in no way worshiping them in any religious sense. We know that they were mortal men and walked the Earth as human beings. They were involved in both the good and the bad that men do. They were not perfect and should not be treated as such.

They did, however, achieve a level of proficiency, and their greatness continues down into you. Just as you may not have met your great-grandfather or great-grandmother, part of them is in you; their nose or their eyes sit on your face, looking at you daily in the mirror.

It is said that the martial arts begin and end with respect. Our place of practice is a special place. It is the space where your metamorphosis will take place. It is on the mats where your soul and the souls of countless others will lock horns and clash in endless rounds of live sparring, rolling, grappling, and more. It is the place where you can renew yourself after a 9 to 5 shift and a terrible day or after a rude customer put you in a bad mood. All of your outside problems will vanish for a time, and your spirit or childlike nature will arise because you will be engaged in learning and improving. This is particularly true in Jiujitsu, as you are always faced with a problem that you must solve.

You are playing this physical game of chess during which you will be forced to journey inward and face the real you, not the illusion of you trapped in the daily material social matrix. The courtesy shown before stepping on the mats and leaving the mats is not mandatory in many schools; often I will be the only one doing it. Then suddenly, a superstar such as George St. Pierre or Lyoto Machida will come to visit. They naturally bow before entering the mats, and soon others want to imitate.

What many do not understand is that the bow comes from within. It comes from what is called kokoro, or heart. It is not done as a show or means of approval.

I can recall the first time I bowed to the sword in Iaido practice. There was an overwhelming sense of gratitude and falling away of ego. This sense of inner joy came from the correction that sword practice will do to you. Even a very advanced martial artist will be shocked at how off he is in terms of angle, stance, breath, precision, grip, etc. Through picking up the katana under the wisdom of a good teacher, you will see and deeply respect all these things. If we journey further, we will see the furnace, the blacksmith's den—a place for forging the steel at about 1,150 degrees Celsius, the great heat necessary for the hot forging of steel.

Therefore, the blacksmith's den is an extremely hot place where hours and days are spent hammering the steel together, and heating it folding it, heating it, beating it over and over again, allowing the steel to combine, shaping it, molding it, engineering it towards perfection. The interesting thing about Japanese steel is its composition of various types of metals—one of a strong nature, and one of a flexible kind.

The forging process will not only combine these metals to give the steel unmatched toughness, but it will also remove impurities.

This removal of impurities is the same thing that happens to you once you begin training on the mats. What are your impurities? Your fear, your doubt, your hesitation, your impatience, your anger, your lack of self-confidence, your overconfidence, etc.?

You also will be molded into a priceless treasure, a wonderful human being, and a person of a sturdy heart. You will become a keeper of the way. Yes, there will be countless swords that break under that pressure and do not make it out of the blacksmith's den. But, for those that can take the heat, hone the edge, and be placed in the hands of a worthy swordsman, it is a blessing supreme.

So you see, if we use only the naked eye, we would look in an empty room and say, "Why is that guy bowing to the mats?" But when we journey inward, through an in-depth perception, we see that he is not bowing to vinyl and foam mats, woven soft rush straw, tatami, or hardwood floors. He is entering into the correct mind space for learning, emptying his cup, and connecting to the tradition of respect that has been passed down throughout the generations.

To bow to the mats or your training partner does not make you invincible. In fact, in the confines of a sparring session, the young man who knows nothing of the martial art tradition but who is a Division I wrestler will most likely send the traditional martial artist to the canvas headfirst.

He does not know of this word "reiho"; he knows only hard work, repetition, and mat time. Seen in this way, it would be easy to dismiss the courtesy. However, the view is the main thing. That is the correct view. Fighting and combat are only one branch of the large martial arts tree. I will keep reminding you of the correct view because I know that your ego is a formidable opponent and will not simply give in. Meditation has an interesting function. Sometimes it can make you become more of your deeper emotions because you can connect better.

So, if you are inwardly angry or internally upset, sometimes connecting to the deeper you can bring those thoughts or emotions to the surface quicker. The same goes for a happy person who loves laughter.

It is the "angry drunk" syndrome. The alcohol did not make this person suddenly become angry. The alcohol simply allowed the normal defensive measures to take a break, to relax. These defensive soldiers protect you. They prevent others from seeing your genuine thoughts and emotions.

This does not mean alcohol is the new meditation. Ultimately, it is an external pleasure, one that is outside you. On the other hand, meditation is you, only you. In my old dojo we had a kanji scroll on the wall, that read, "Extract the essence, and distill it."

That kanji contained a very profound truth to good Budo practice. That is, first to extract, or to bring forward, so the emotions you are hiding will be extracted, brought to the surface, no matter what they are. That is because on the mats, you cannot hide. The second part is to distill, or, in this case, to vaporize, to bring to a state of purification, a state of nothingness and non-attachment.

The correct view in Budo must go beyond yourself or beyond you winning or losing a tournament. A technique is good, but it is similar to technology. At one time cassettes were the way to go, then there were CDs, and now there is streaming. What will be next? Although the technology has advanced and updated, what remains is the voice, the rhythm, the seed.

Do not make the mistake of comparing flowers with seeds. There will always be a way to enhance a new technique, but a principle lasts a lifetime and beyond. Thus, our reiho is a seed. If grown inwardly, it will produce an outward victory to the principle of honor.

This bow towards the mats, this simple gesture, encompasses the bringing together of mind, body, breath, and soul to remember that all that we do on the mats should bring honor to our training partners and to the masters. The mats are not the mats of a gym or a health club where idle talk, gossip, and folly are accepted. The mats reside in a special place—a dojo, a place of the way 道.

So then what is that way? It is a pathless path that ultimately leads you to the best version of you. When you show courtesy to the mats, you ready your mind's eye for learning. The important thing is that we set the example so future generations will look toward this. Then, after a hard session, they will sweep and clean the mats—cleaning what looks like the outer hall but is actually the inner.

If the place is a place of the way, you will know it. You will feel it, it will be difficult to go on or off the mats without being moved to make a silent bow. The training and tutelage will have pierced your ego. The ego will humbly bow and allow the space for your mind's eye to learn and grow in Budo, and you will come upon that which is timeless. As it is said, "Collect yourself, then enter."

This understanding is for those who intend to be warriors.

4

Take Ukemi/Be a Uke

*"If you slip in the streets,
you gotta take your falls, Osu!"*
—Soke Lil John Davis—

I am not sure what came first. The sound or the fury after the lightning speed throw that I received from Kaicho, Soke Lil John Davis. At a workshop on Sanuces Ryu Jiujitsu, he asked me to feed him a reverse punch and, upon deflecting my strike and securing a Kote-Gaeshi with tai otoshi leg, he looked back at me with a smile and said, "You got your falls?" I replied, "Osu!"

Then, within the blink of an eye, I had break-falled on the mat. I will say without a doubt that what I had received from that one throw from Master Lil John Davis was worth a trillion martial arts lessons, an infinite amount of wisdom in speed, timing, sensitivity, and power. It is interesting that in all throws, there is a sense of being in the air, even if it is a fraction of a second. You can feel yourself going up and then coming down. However, on that day, the throw I felt was different, like none other, even to this day.

It was as if we were connected, he smiled, then we were disconnected. I got up and we embraced as brothers. What an honor to be thrown by that great man. It had taken some time to even understand what had happened that day. Then, on a rainy afternoon, it all made sense. In Zen training, a senior abbot will give a trainee a koan.

A koan is like a riddle with no logical answer. For example, "What is the sound of one hand clapping?" or "How do you hit the center of a circle?" These koans are designed to almost frustrate the mind, to make the mind's eye expand and move away from the trappings of the logical mind. It is a difficult task. In the average mind, 2+2 should be 4. However, in the Zen mind, you are the sum of all things, yet nothing. So 2+2 may or may not be 4.

In the mind of most, when a strike is thrown and the master performs some move, a first thought is, "Would that work?" or "Would that work in a street fight?" We are concentrating on the finger pointing away to the moon, so we miss all the heavenly glory.

It was on a rainy afternoon that I had watched my favorite martial arts documentary titled *The Warrior Within.* There was a section of the documentary that featured Soke Lil John's teacher, the late Doctor Moses Powell. In this section, Master Lil John was the uke, he was receiving ukemi from his teacher, taking fall after fall and technique after technique, all with highly evident pain yet fluidity and grace.

It was at that moment that I understood what it means to receive ukemi or to be a uke. I understood why his throw was so unique. It was simple: It was not the throw of one man. It was the technique passed from grandmaster to master, and from master to student, along with countless shiai experiences of his own, and more. So, in essence, it was a single throw with the wisdom and experience of a hundred men.

To be a uke for the master is a high honor. You get real-time, first-hand experience directly from the teacher's hand. All of his feeling is slowly passed down to you, literally directly into your bloodstream.

The master's years of sacrifice to refine his motion are handed down to you, like a gift.

It is still on you to receive that gift. In order to fully receive these gifts of feeling, the uke must empty his cup to receive the herbal benefits of the master's tea.

There was a swordsman who traveled a long and difficult road up the steep mountain. His intentions were to bring his swordsmanship to the next level. It was known that a master teacher had lived in the upper mountain. Upon arrival, the teacher had asked the man to come in and sit. The young man, being eager and ready, did not wish to sit. He wanted to start right away. The master said, "Let's first have some tea."

The young man obliged and sat. And before the master could say anything, the young man began to talk about a few of his specialties. He began to explain the techniques that he favored, the methods he thought worked and others that he felt did not work. He also began to let the master know that he was proficient in various ryuha and also understood the fundamentals of the master's ryu, which was of the Ko Ryu Kenjutsu. The master smiled and poured tea for himself first. Then he began pouring tea for the young swordsman.

Although the tea began to reach the top of the cup, the master continued to pour, and the tea overflowed onto the table, then down to the floor, creating a big mess as the master continued to pour.

The swordsman was shocked by this, and he leaped out of his chair, yelling, "What are you doing?" The master replied, "Young man, your cup overflows. You must learn to empty it."

There is a process of emptying your cup. There is an inward humbling that must occur to your ego. For some, this is natural, but for others it is so difficult. In Budo, the flower can be seen as a metaphor for the importance of not outward beauty, but for inborn growth, which leads to an outward beauty.

I can recall during Jiujitsu practice pairing up with a man who was at a blue belt rank when I was already a brown belt. It was not odd for a higher rank to work with or train with a lower-ranking student. What was odd was that this particular student had been training at the academy for just as long as, if not longer than, me. How could he still be at the blue belt level? I saw him weekly, and he even sat closer to the professor as techniques were being taught. How could this be? He had not been injured or spent any time away from the mats. So then, what was it?

Fate would have it that on that day, we would be paired together to work with each other to repeat the techniques that the professor had taught. It was there that it all came together.

This training session was done without the gi. Therefore, we did not wear our belt rank. As I started to perform the technique upon him, me being the tori, he immediately was not being a good uke. He was resisting and countering or trying to counter each technique that was being taught.

Then, when we switched roles and he was the tori, he basically forgot the techniques because, in his mind, he was too occupied with countering the moves that were taught. His cup was so full he was never able to taste the master's tea. This inability to humble oneself to learn shares a distant cousin, it is the same trap that does not allow you to see the energy, flow, and direction of a technique and causes you to ask instead, "Would that work?" It is the formless, mischievous one. It is the ego.

There, under all your logic and reason, sits the troublemaker waiting, blocking, and hindering your every chance to gain a deeper insight. You could be physically so close to the teacher yet be the furthest away from his teachings.

I cannot recall the first time I was called up to be a uke for my teacher. It was long ago. I do remember, however, being very excited. I knew that my teacher did not just call up anybody, it had to be someone who could flow well. Again, remember the metaphor of the flower and its beauty. The technique is not trying to look beautiful. However, when tori and uke move together, it is the most beautiful thing an eye can see. It is like a dance of death that produces life.

The onlooking student should have a sense of inspiration to better himself or herself to attain that level of fluidity. The uke has a very big role, more important than he or she knows. Ukes also teach. They teach the onlooking student how to receive the tori's energy. They show how to receive directional force and how to move with the movement or resist movement depending on the technique at hand.

You may then think that the uke will improve or excel at a faster rate than others. The answer is absolutely yes, if they are willing to empty their cup and be awake to the feeling. I have seen and felt this first-hand.

My professor, John Danaher, was once called John New Zealand, and our first encounter was a memorable one. My training partners were all raving about this man named Big John, or John New Zealand. He is a student of the legendary Renzo Gracie.

While being uke for Professor Danaher, my training partner, whose name also was John, had been literally put to sleep during the teaching of a technique. This happens through no error of the tori. This is a rare occurrence in which the uke does not tap in time.

The precision of choking techniques has an interesting effect. When done correctly, a blood choke can become more comfortable, not painful. So comfortable, in fact, you may even take a nap.

So off to the academy John and I went. After Professor Renzo Gracie taught, everyone stayed around for randori, or live grappling matches. This was a No-Gi practice session. Thus, no one knew each other's rank. At that time, Professor John was a brown belt, and I had just received my blue belt.

As we started rolling, I was immediately met by an entirely different feeling altogether. I instantly knew I was in the presence of a master. In Jiujitsu there is often a feeling from beginner to high intermediate practitioners of speed, strength, untamed pressure, and a chaining together of attempted techniques.

What there is not a feeling of is slow motion, Tai Chi–like control. Being that I was already a student in Yang–style Tai Chi, I was very keen on what proper breathing and correct sensitivity should feel like.

Professor John used total body sensitivity to control my every movement, and I was very impressed by this level of technical proficiency. He was using two principles: leverage and simplicity. I can only describe our first training session as being buried alive in sand or sakrete, which is a heavier grade of sand that turns into concrete.

Later, when I found out who he was, he humbly smiled. It is an interesting thing to note that some of the most skilled, deadly practitioners of the art are the most humble, ego-less, down-to-earth individuals on the planet. Professor John had used various ukes, depending on class schedule and availability; early morning would be Boris, the afternoon would be Shawn Williams. One uke began to emerge as a very consistent uke for Professor John. That was Brian Glick.

Again, the metaphor of the flower emerges. It is not trying to look beautiful but, because of the cycles of nature's nurturing, the flower grows into a thing of beauty. So, if it is nature and its cycles that produce the beauty of the flower, then it is the sky–like view and compassion of the teacher that produce the polished skills of the student.

In Kung Fu there is what is called a signature hand, a distinctive identity to a hand that only the educated eye can see. In Japan, we can also see this in waza variations. While some Judo schools may prefer a particular grip, any exponent of Koga Judo will have a unique grip on uchimata based on their teacher Toshihiko Koga. Thus, your lineage is of importance.

It was indeed a beautiful thing to see and feel Mr. Glick's progression over the years. Not only did his Jiujitsu level improve, but I noticed a particular signature feeling emerging: He felt more and more like his teacher, moving more smoothly and tactically with each passing year.

Budo is indeed a peculiar thing. We on the mats or in the dojo are not related by DNA, yet we share chromosomes of the teacher through attitude and sensitivity. So, the name "dojo" or "place of the way," could not be more fitting. So then, the way becomes an important thing when we see those who are not of the way exploiting people's fears or lack of understanding and teaching gimmick martial arts: I blow on you, you get knocked down, I punch four feet away from you, and all three students get sent to the ground in pain. I use my ki to protect my body from blunted spears, or I simply stare at you and you are incapacitated.

These things are not the way. They are gimmicks and should be looked at as such. However, it does speak to the wanting in mankind.

Once, my Sifu Ralph Mitchell and I attended an excellent Wing Chun workshop. The instructor had flown in all the way from California. He was highly skilled, his speed was a sight to behold, and we worked on close-quarter combat and tactics of Wing Chun chi sao, or sticking hands—a great workshop indeed.

However, at the end of the workshop, the teacher began talking about Shin Kung, which is spiritual Kung Fu. He said that through a particular set of breathing patterns, he would be able to uproot a practitioner who was in their stance and move them without touching them. "Impossible," I thought. "There is no way he can move them without touching them. It is absolute rubbish."

One by one, he went down the line and, without touching each student, he began a series of deep breaths, sweating, and deep concentration. To my surprise, each beginner student was moving off balance slightly, either stepping back or forward to regain their lost balance. But I was still highly skeptical and not a believer.

My Sifu Ralph Mitchell stood next to me in the line. I had committed myself to absolutely become a believer if the teacher could move my Sifu. Then, their eyes met. The Wing Chun teacher was shaking, sweating, attempting with all and every ounce of concentrated power to move my Sifu. The teacher was turning red, muscles straining, fingers tightening, teeth clenching, eyes focusing, legs trembling. However, it did not work. It failed, and failed miserably. Seeing that I was a student of Sifu, he did not try that on me. He simply gave us a thumbs up and said, "Good Kung Fu."

Later I asked Sifu, "Did you feel anything? Could he have possibly moved you?" Sifu replied, "If I was any less centered, I could have been moved. Some people 'want to be moved.'"

How does it occur that the beginner uke later becomes a skilled intermediate and, one day, a master teacher himself? It is the simplest yet hardest thing to do. Empty the cup, be as an empty boat, and allow the stream to move you where it will.

The good uke will not only pick up mannerisms of the tori, but he will also have an insight into the attitude behind the technique or task at hand and develop a similar touch of the master. He will be able to decipher good energy from bad. He will ultimately become a teacher himself. Then, one day, he will call someone forward, some unsuspecting student. That student will have the honor of being his uke, and he will take ukemi. Thus is the circle of Budo.

This understanding is for those who intend to be warriors.

5
Fold Your Gi

*"The purpose of training is to tighten up the slack,
toughen up the body and polish the spirit."*
—Morihei Ueshiba—

I took my training partner to the side. I told him with the utmost sincerity and compassion that his gi stunk and that was probably why no one wanted to grapple with him. There is, of course, the usual stench of sweat, blood, and mildew of hot and humid bodies. That is a normal thing on the mats. This, however, was a special case. After our brief conversation, he said, "This is the only gi I have. I have been wearing it for weeks."

I took him in the locker room, opened my dojo bag, and gave him my spare gi. He was shocked by the gesture. But he was more shocked that the gi was folded, wrapped by an obi, clean, and ready to be employed.

Often, it is a common thing to simply throw the gi in your training bag before practice, and throw it back in after practice with little or any care to its order. In comparison to technical ability, folding your uniform would, unfortunately, rank very low in the mind of the practitioner.

However, if we go deeper, if we begin to journey inward, we will see that folding your gi is much more than a mundane chore. It is part of an essential skill set and will give you sight beyond sight. It will give you insight.

In combat, we have stances, or postures (kamae). In Thai boxing, the stance is designed to utilize the legs to deliver explosive, rapid-fire kicks and to deliver powerful knees or elbows. In boxing, the stance, or kamae, is designed to protect the upper body while delivering punishing blows to an opponent. In Judo, the stance is designed to maintain balance while off-balancing your opponent, then being able to enter, fit, and take your opponent down to score ippon.

In ancient times, there were various restrictions on the behavior of samurai: ways of standing, sitting, bowing, and walking, ways of turning corners and leaving or entering a room, and even more guidelines for behavior upon arrival at the destination. A true samurai was always on the threshold of life and death, so he could not show unpreparedness or careless openings to an opponent.

With the sword, some various postures or stances allow for attack and defense. There are, however, hidden stances, inward stances, such as ki gamae or kokoro gamae. There is also sight—interpretive sight (egen), neutral perspective (tengen), the naked eye (nikugan), compassionate eye (shingan/higan), and the compelling insight.

The etiquette of Budo is not merely good manners. Every action of protocol indicates the possibility of a sudden attack. Thus, it includes a posture for defense and counter. The correct internalization must be prepared inwardly first so that one is outwardly ready.

On one winter morning, as I prepared for Zen and Iaido practice, the dojo was freezing as usual. Everyone was pushing through the cold and putting on their gis, which felt like ice on the skin. My senpai was about to put on his hakama. But, before he did so, he pointed to the interweaving, folded pattern in the himo and how the fold should be able to be undone with simply one pull.

I asked him, "Why was that necessary?" He replied, "For quick access, in case we have to man our stations or defend intrusion." It was then that I made a great connection. Although we are in the 21st century and our dojos are not being invaded like Osaka Castle during the Summer Siege in 1614. There was something of a deep connection to the ready mind state, to see the training beyond the physical push-pull and tactical theory.

But, to be ready! To hear the words of the master in a ready state is where much more saturation occurs.

If my hakama, or gi, was not folded after sword practice, the unfolded cloth would remain in the bag. Upon opening the bag, I would immediately know on such and such day that I was in a rush, careless. It was a strong reminder to be present at all times and to truly attend.

According to Yamamoto Tsunetomo, it is good to carry some powdered rouge in one's sleeve. It may happen that when one is sobering up or waking from sleep, his complexion may be poor. At such a time, it is good to take out and apply some powdered rouge.

These stories point to preparedness, which comes from the simple act of folding your gi. It points to what my senpai said about being ready. It points beyond martial arts—it points to martial living. It is simple: You can train as a hobbyist, just to physically move and maintain the body as exercise, to win a competition, or to achieve other goals.

However, the wine will be finished and the music track will cease. Then, what will you be left with? Silence. The folding of the gi has very little to do with being neat. However, it is refreshing to have a clean, fresh gi to put on for each session, as it will help your mind become new and set a good physical and mental stage for learning. Also, your training partners will be happy to roll with you because you do not smell of a rotten cesspool.

So, the outer is a byproduct of the more critical aspects that make up martial living: preparing the gi with care, carefully detailing it, and getting your mind and spirit ready for the next session.

This will begin to overflow into other areas of life. You will foresee traffic, you will leave earlier, you will arrive on time. You will be diligent with your weapons, never careless; you will tend to unfinished business; you will be a martial professional. Then it will become a good habit and you will lead by example.

Upon my arrival at the Kodokan in Japan, the interesting thing was that none of the Judokas spoke English, or very little at most. But we all spoke Judo, which is kuzushi, tsukuri, an ippon. We can also say elevation, rotation, and impact.

It was a great experience in which there was no wine, no music, or even the ability to communicate with standard language. We communicated through the language of Budo, blood, sweat (a lot of sweat), and tears. I can recall that after training I folded my gi and used my obi to tie it and carry it shoulder–style. As the highest-ranking members watched me naturally fold my gi and hoist it over my shoulder, they looked on with smiles of appreciation, for they had seen the unseen.

According to what one of the Judo elders said, there are seven disciplines associated with diligent training:

1. Avoid falsehood in spirit
2. Do not lose confidence
3. Correct your posture
4. Be swift
5. Use your power without restraint
6. Do not neglect your training
7. Discipline yourself

If we look at the seventh principle, discipline yourself, we can see how crucial it is to remember, even though it may seem a bit vague or grand in nature. Disciplining yourself lies at the center of all that we are as warriors. Discipline is the string that holds all mala beads together.

Just as a chain is only as strong as its weakest link, so too is your discipline. Whatever areas you favor often get more attention. Similar to the bodybuilder who exclusively focuses on upper body training, there will be an imbalance at the core of even the simplest technique.

This discipline can make you become an expert at a particular technique. If you work at it diligently day in and day out and hit countless correct repetitions, you will master the subtleties of timing, making the technique look effortless. There will be no gap between you and the technique. If the opponent's foot is misplaced, you will sweep him. If the opponent strikes, you will evade. The natural simplicity of the flow of your action comes by way of discipline.

So the seventh principle, discipline yourself, means to put forth discipline in everything you do, including cooking a meal, making your bed, being on time for a meeting, training in any art or craft, and absolutely taking care of your uniform. Just as in Judo, the essence is to not lose your center. You also must not lose the center of discipline in all actions. This does not mean you are perfect. It does mean, however, you have a perfect plan.

In a state of being unshakable, steady, aware, and awake in nage waza, if we lose our center, we get thrown. If we land on our back, it is ippon; we have lost. Compare this to an argument. Someone said something, pissed you off, you lost your cool, lost your center, took actions, or said something you regret. You lost. It is over. A relationship is ruined, a friendship is gone, time is lost. When our center is imbalanced, we will fall. Also, the opposite holds true. When we keep our center, we remain victorious. Using a sky–like view, when others attempt to off-balance your center, it is a difficult task because your level of discipline has trained the eye to see incipient actions at all levels. You have obtained a potent tool: insight. You can see something for what it is and not what it appears to be.

You are everywhere protected, as you have become the seventh principle: you are disciplined. The discipline of the mind is the basic ingredient for genuine morality and spiritual strength. When you journey inward and shine the light of discipline into every area of your being, you will see that taking care of your gi would never be something separate from you. The gi is you. You are the gi.

This understanding is for those who intend to be warriors.

6

Step into the Ring

"You must have a dragon hidden inside you.
When you need, you let the dragon out."
—Anderson Silva—

"Get out of your comfort zone," were the words that Sifu always said. It meant not to stagnate, not to achieve a way and say "this is the way." Our path in Budo is a path toward truth, toward an ultimate principle. Truth is a pathless land.

Sure, there are steps, a directive, instructions, and a guide that go with most endeavors. Learn the steps, follow the steps, adhere to the directive, then, ultimately, dissolve the lessons.

As a teenager, I can recall meeting Guru Dan Inosanto for the first time. He was a direct student of the late Li Shiao Long (Bruce Lee). I recall after a six hour workshop, we were all exhausted. We had covered in depth the art of Pangamut (Filipino boxing) and Kali. After our workshop, I remember shaking his hand for the first time. He said two words that were shocking to hear.

He had taught with tremendously detailed instruction, exact directives for close-quarter combat, and much more. I felt I owed him so much for dropping so many precious gemstones. Then, upon leaving and shaking my hand, he simply smiled and said, "Thank you."

How could a man of such stature and martial arts status thank me? I felt it was I who should have been thanking him. It was at that very moment that I had a grand awakening about the spirit of a good martial artist. I realized that great skill and technique can be achieved by many, but humbleness only by a few.

Guru Dan proceeded to sign my book (written by his teacher), *The Tao of Jeet Kune Do*. My Sifu said the important thing was to "become the book" beyond the written words, to dissolve the message into your soul.

You see, the instructions are good. However, they are also a confinement, a sort of box that we can get caught in or a comfort zone that we can get used to, a set schedule that we adhere to religiously, a gospel truth that cannot be changed.

There is a way to transcend the words and truly see the spirit of a thing. And that is to put it to the test. The correlation between your shadow boxing and bag work should be seamless.

Your practice is similar to the lanes of a highway and can be seen as such. The destination you seek can be achieved by either lane. However, the speed and rhythm of each lane are dramatically different. Thus, respect for each lane is necessary. Everyone has their own strengths, weaknesses, coordination, personality, etc. Those traits are what determine the lane you drive in.

The understanding of lanes as a metaphor is essential. It will instantly put into the perspective the joy of learning. Your ego will begin to stand at ease. Once you start lane comparison, you will realize the error in comparing a young man of age nineteen who has few responsibilities to a father of three children who owns and operates a hectic business, or a shy teenager who has been bullied to a teenager who is the captain of the football team and a star athlete.

The lanes are essential. They give you what is called the "correct view," just as in martial arts, a high achievement will be the rank called the black belt. We will arrive there in different ways and at different times. It is important to see that, as we train and prepare, we each are going our way, similar to the lanes of a highway, yet we are moving or flowing together as a stream. Some move up, some move down, and others move in East–West patterns. It is simple. It is the path of learning. That is it.

So the question arises, How do we make the vehicle as efficient as possible? How do we ensure its function during real-time hardships such as storms, steep hills, slippery surfaces, or sharp turns? How do we ensure that the driver of such a vehicle has adaptability and experience to face such hardships? There is only one way. Put the vehicle to the test, a test to ensure that all systems are functioning, including the internal workings, such as suspension, transmission, etc.

A racetrack and a highway both have lanes. However, there is a difference on a large scale. On a racetrack, you are all moving and competing to reach the finish line. There is a clear goal to reach, and there are rules and regulations for meeting such goals.

You are bound, bound by a particular rule set to achieve your goal and cross the finish line faster than everyone else on the track. It is in this very strict set of rules, which one has to adhere to in order to be the victor, where actually a greater freedom arises. In order to see this freedom or to attain it, you must journey inward.

According to the way of the samurai, a meditation on one's own death should be performed daily. Every day, when one's mind and body are at peace, one should meditate on being carried away by a great wave or falling from a thousand-foot cliff, being ripped apart by arrows and spears, being shaken to death by a great earthquake, dying of disease, being thrown into the midst of a great fire, being struck by lightning, or committing seppuku at the death of one's own master and, every day without fail, one should consider himself as dead.

To the naked eye or ear, this could appear like a horrible thought, something that we are all frightened of. On the contrary, it is the most liberating state of mind to be in, free of any doubt, fear, or hesitation. It is the mind state of the victorious. So how can it be that dying inwardly can free you outwardly? First, we have to understand the context of death. For now, we will understand death as an ending. An ending of a time. An ending of a relationship, an ending of an obligation, or an ending of a moment.

This ending gives us two fundamental aspects to look at. First, at the time of the end, what has been left behind? What memory did we leave, what lives did we touch, what joy did we bring, what pain did we bring, did we leave the legacy we intended, will what we left behind help or hurt the world?

Second, knowing that this death is coming, did you fully live? Did you truly cherish the people in your life, did you hear and apply the wisdom of the elders? Did you settle affairs, did you observe the inner beauty of nature, have you stood still in the breeze, have you lived each day fully and wholeheartedly with few regrets, have you taken the time to say what needs to be said to those you care for and others in the world?

It is this correct view of death that teaches us not to be frightened of death, including the physical end, and not to be a slave to the arrival of death. It teaches us to not take things for granted.

I can recall one of my boxing coaches, the late George Washington of Bed–Stuy boxing gym, a veteran of WWII, and a boxing southpaw genius. He would sit in front of the gym, always looking out the window at passersby. His eye, however, was keen on exactly what you were doing on the heavy bag.

He would yell and shout from his chair without leaving his seat and create champions. Every Thursday, like clockwork, was our training time. It was he who taught me how to wrap hands for boxing. Our routine was the same. Upon entry, George, as he liked to be called, would take my hand wraps and meticulously wrap each hand, first the left hand, then the right. Next, it was on to shadow boxing and ring work. He and my uncle, Clarence Benyard, would fire away commands. "When you step back, don't step all the way back, step short," he would yell. Or, "When you throw your power shot, bring the hook back!"

These words of instruction always echoed through the gym and still echo in me today. After ring work, we would go to either heavy bag work or sparring, and that was where the magic would happen. He and my uncle, "Uncle Bernie," had a way of creating an atmosphere of actual combat in which you hit the heavy bag. I was not simply striking the heavy bag as most do today. It was a fight.

They pushed me mentally to visualize the bag as an actual opponent that I could never slack off from while in front of, or disrespect by punching sluggishly or, the cardinal sin, dropping my hands. He pushed me to journey inward and connect the dots of power, speed, and accuracy to the mind's eye of an actual opponent, not a large, leather bag filled with sand or other materials but an actual person with whom I was always in a state of opposition. My knuckles, although wrapped, would still feel sore after striking with every ounce to rip through the core of the bag.

After about eight intense rounds, I would finish with conditioning. The jump rope was saved for last, along with crunches.

All along, George would simply watch, not yell, just observe my level of determination, or lack thereof. Finally, he would unravel my hand wraps, shake my hand, and we would repeat the following week.

I will never forget the day I went to the gym and George was not present. When I asked, they said he was not feeling too well. Shortly after, George passed away. He was gone. Just like that, a man of such generosity and sincere love had transitioned to join the ancestors. Initially, there was a heavy silence, a deep feeling of sorrow from everyone.

When I passed the window of the gym, it was so painful not to see him sitting in the reflection, looking on.

As time went on and I continued training, I could still hear his voice constantly motivating me, pushing me through the rounds. It was then that I realized that the words of the master will forever live on in the student. So, the important thing is to listen.

His passing gave me more intensity in my training; the power now had a purpose. The purpose was to make the words of the teacher become whole. Although physically he was gone, his spirit remained. It was with every breath and every step inside the ring.

The preparation for a competition is a special thing. To succeed, it is important to know your opponent, but the more important thing is to know yourself. Not only do you need to see the result of giving your best punch or kick in sparring, but you must also know where your head is at when you receive someone's best punch or kick. Did their strike make you angry, did you lose focus, did you feel an overwhelming desire for revenge, or did you get excited and return a sadistic smile?

These emotions that hide within us all must be brought to the surface prior to stepping into a competition. Bringing your emotions to the surface is vital to knowing yourself. In stepping in the ring, there is nowhere to hide, not even from yourself. Often my students have told me or, rather, complained that the training for the tournament is much harder than the tournament itself. I answer with, "That is why your hand will be raised in victory."

The win, lose, or draw in the competition is the secondary win. The first victory is to win inwardly, to conquer and make friends with all your emotions, including the bottom dwellers, such as doubt and fear. It would be wrong to see the competition stage only as an actual tournament, with promoters, officials, etc. Instead, you should see any endeavor in which you set forward to excel as your personal competition stage. So, when you are faced with opposition, you will remember the words of the master to not hurt another, but to maximize your potential. Maximizing your potential requires looking within yourself at every corner and, most importantly, facing your fears.

I can recall when I used to do roadwork in Brooklyn, New York. I would jog the entire length of Ocean Parkway, from the top near Prospect Park all the way to the bottom in Coney Island. There was a large cemetery called the Washington Cemetery that I always had to pass. My roadwork was always done very early in the morning, often before the sun came up. My biggest fear during the competition was the fear of getting tired in a fight. I experienced that once during a San Shou bout and vowed to never feel that way again.

I can recall in that bout that both my opponent and I were dead tired in the final round. I had to summon every ounce of my being to push forward. I secured his back and threw him over my head with a back suplex. That was my "one more action with certainty," which led to victory. However, I will never forget the feeling of being fatigued, my mind still strong, still pushing forward, but my body too exhausted to follow through. It is like a nightmare, except you are fully awake and it is real.

As I jogged down the lengthy streets of Ocean Parkway, when I passed the cemetery, it was my landmark to keep pushing forward. I could still hear the words of the master from beyond the grave, telling me to keep pushing and keep running forward.

It is a fact that the words of the master will continue to be the wind under your wings as you soar to new heights and progress as a human being, a father, a brother, a businessman, a competitor. There is a sense of giri (obligation) to the master, a remembrance of the master's sacrifice of time, energy, and care to see you improve. It will always result in your putting forth your best effort, your most sincere ability.

At the heart of all competition-based endeavors is the question of whose ability can surpass all the others, and whose prowess can excel. When the ego has been humbled through preparation to step into the ring, we see clearly that a special thing has occurred. We have fortified our potential, brought honor to the master, had life in every breath, and prepared to die a glorious death.

This understanding is for those who intend to be warriors.

7
Clean the Blade

"The sword is the soul.
Study the sword to know the soul."
—Dai-bosatsu Tōge—

According to what one of the elders said, if you are handling a sharp knife, you must have a steady hand.

In Iaido (Japanese swordsmanship) practice during Kata, there are a few essential points that permeate all Kata. That is, the quick drawing of the sword, a sharp cut with a clear line, a shaking off of the sword we call chiburi, a resheathing of the sword we call noto, and a closure while remaining in a state of zanshin, or total awareness within a lingering heart.

Iaido is indeed a unique form of Budo. It requires a certain level of maturity, a particular awareness as you practice, a connection between the breath and the movements of the sword that gives life to the sword, and tremendous attention to detail. My teacher, Robert Savoca Sensei, embodies all of these things. One of our warm-ups every practice was called suburi. In suburi practice, we repeatedly swing the sword in a large motion down the center line in a stable yet deep stance while counting aloud. It builds up good stamina of the body, breath, and mind. Suburi training, when done properly, will also take you on a journey inward. It was always a beautiful thing to see Sensei Savoca cutting effortlessly. His cutting always made me remember the warlord Takeda Shingen's battle flag—swift like the wind, gentle like a forest, fierce like the fire, and unshakable like a mountain.

In sword practice, there are only two things we cut. One is the air. The other is some type of cutting target, which can range from tatami omote to bamboo to other things such as animal carcasses. I would recommend sticking to tatami omote. When cutting targets, the shinken passes through the material. This material will cling to the sword. If left uncleaned, it can leave rust deposits on the blade and ultimately ruin the sword. So, for obvious reasons, after cutting practice (tameshigiri), the sword should always be cleaned, polished, oiled, etc.

During Kata practice, however, the sword is cutting only through air. To the naked eye, there is nothing on the blade, no visible particles—maybe a little dust—but basically not much. Then why even clean the blade at all?

First, it is a good habit to form, as there are unseen moisture particles that can cling to the sword, especially when many people are in practice on a humid day. But let us go deeper. When you polish the sword, you polish your soul. To clean the blade, you use a few essential items. In a basic cleaning kit, you will usually have a cloth, a small hammer to remove the mekugi, a uchiko-powder ball, and choji oil. You will then need well-lit, ample space, as well as an area to place the saya. Have you ever been walking down the street when something suddenly got in your eye? For those few seconds, the whole world stopped. You instantly sent all your forces on a mission, a mission to clear your vision and rid your eye of the intruder.

When you clean the sword, for that moment all other traffic in your mind should disperse. As you begin to focus in on the sword, you will start to move meticulously: carefully coating the blade with uchiko powder, slowly bringing the sword to its original luster.

I have had a collection of martial arts weapons since I was young, mostly from Kung Fu—the staff, spear, trident, three-sectional staff, kwan-do, tiger hooks, cudgel, rope dart, and, my favorite, the steel whip.

I was determined to gain proficiency in all of these weapons. Each of these weapons can teach you a lot about body connection and mobility because the weapon should not be separate from you—it should be an extension of you. You and the weapon must become one.

During my quest for weapon art, I learned the art of Kali (a Filipino martial art), and it was in the Filipino arts that my weapon training became functional.

The art is focused on lightning speed combinations with the Escrima stick and close-quarter combat with the knife, a tactical endeavor for sure. My Sifu Ralph Mitchell's words always echoed in my head. He said, "Functionalize your art and do well what you do well."

My next rite of passage in weapon art was to actually fight with the weapons. So I entered full-contact stick-fighting tournaments. In these fights, we wore headgear and body armor. However, when the stick is unleashed with full power, you can absolutely feel the impact. Instead of trophies being awarded at one particular tournament, the Doce Pares family decided to award us with actual swords. Third place received a dagger, second place received a kris, and first place received a barong (Filipino leaf blade).

I recall the final match after I had beat everyone in my division. I was determined to win the barong, as it was the only weapon that I did not have in my collection. The morning before the tournament, I was up early practicing and getting ready for battle. I had envisioned using a particular uppercut strike used by my Sifu in the past.

Although we wore gloves, the entire forearm was exposed. During a furious exchange, I caught a full power blow to the forearm. The pain cut right through to the bone. However, I remained intact, continuously moving forward and overwhelming my opponent with a barrage of strikes from every possible angle conceivable. I was able to land the famous uppercut and disarm my opponent. It was a victorious day. Indeed, I was able to bring home the first prize: the barong.

When I brought the barong home, I was so elated. It joined my collection of weapons and, more importantly, it had been earned through blood, sweat, tears, and sacrifice.

In the arts such as Kung Fu and the Filipino arts, cleaning our weapons was not part of daily practice. It was done, but not at all in the ritual sense of Japanese Iaido.

Many years after I won the barong, I was already fighting professional MMA. A great match I had was with the highly ranked American top team opponent, Raphael Diaz. We fought everywhere, striking range, clinching and grappling. The fight went the distance. As the judges' scores were being read, I knew I was in his territory and he could get the victory. The judges called it a split decision in favor of Diaz.

The same rush of joy that rips through your soul and into the heavens when your hand is raised in victory also rushes down into the bottomless pit in the face of defeat. After a long flight and plenty of time to think, the feeling of letting everyone down seemed impossible to shake. Then, the hungry ghosts began to enter my mind, looking to feast on doubt, anger, and 1,001 "what ifs?"

Then, one of my brothers in Budo, Professor Clarence Everett, who also cornered me in that fight and others, could see my frustration and feel my pain of a loss. As we sat and talked, we spoke of dying well, without regrets or going out in a blaze of glory.

He noticed my many weapons, one of which was the barong. He said, "This is a beautiful sword, you should clean it." The barong that I had won many years before was on the wall, displayed with many other weapons and picking up all sorts of air deposits, dust, etc.

I had some metal polish and attempted to clean some spots out. However, the marks of rust were too stubborn, I did not think they could come out at all. He said, "Wait, let me try." Slowly, little by little, inch by inch, he used small circular motions with steady pressure, attention to detail, and, most importantly, patience. To my surprise, the barong that I cherished so much returned to its original shine. In fact, after oil was applied, it shined even brighter.

We then took out all my blades and weapons. We spent the entire afternoon polishing swords and cleaning blades. They all became like new. My fight with Diaz, the pain of the loss, and the feeling of doubt and frustration all had been totally washed away. It was as though my soul and original mind had been renewed, cleaned, polished, and brought to a place of peace and serenity.

It is something to remember that the sword that kills is the same sword that gives life. However, that sword from time to time must be cleaned. Especially when it is exposed to the world.

The clinging particles are both physical and spiritual. The original mind must be protected, just as the original blade must be protected.

Our senses—touch, smell, taste, hearing, and sight—can sometimes operate as bandits and steal away or cover up our original minds. Be diligent and do not neglect to clean the blade, for sometimes what is unseen can become manifest. Just like a virus, although unseen with the eye, it can attach itself to your system, lie dormant, and then, when ready, show itself and wreak havoc on you and the world. So, too, can impurities cling to our spirit and cause us to err in judgment.

Once, my student stepped up to cut her first mat in what is called tameshigiri, or test cutting. Although in Iaido she was considered a beginner, her first cut was somewhat of an expert cut. She centered the shinken in front of the tatami omote and raised her arms overhead. I can recall that day well, as well as the silence before her cut as everyone was in a moment of anticipation. It was not only her first cut, but she was also the first to step up and cut in the group.

Gripping the sword tightly, she raised it over her head. Then she brought the sword down at full speed in what we call kesa (a diagonal cut). She had achieved a perfect 45-degree angle effortlessly. The blade of that particular sword was extremely sharp; however, good cutting has a lot less to do with the sharpness of the blade and more with proper body mechanics. The sword is an extension of the body, and the body is an extension of the mind. At the time of her first cut, her mind was empty in a sort of mushin, or no mind mental state.

After the first cut was achieved, there was the memory of success, along with an attachment to that success, a goal to be attained. Her next cut started out looking the same, arms raised overhead in jodan and eyes focused. But the cut was a disaster, knocking over the entire stand and sending small tatami pieces flying everywhere. The cut after that paled in comparison to the previous mess; now the sword was stuck halfway through the target. Tatami was hanging everywhere in a chaotic fashion. The perfect first cut she made could not be recreated.

The unseen attachments can work in small degrees. These degrees can be evident in cutting practice. When cutting the air, these degrees can be heard through hasuji (cutting wind). Our training of daily repetition is to fine-tune our awareness in the now, not the previous day, the last loss, the past success, or the future endeavor. The goal is to be present and to, indeed, attend. Not to achieve mushin, but to be mushin.

In battle, it is of the utmost importance to have a clear mind. All that we do is an extension of the mind fueled by the spirit. As we clean the blade, it is renewed, restored, ready to be drawn again. When we polish the sword, we polish the soul.

This understanding is for those who intend to be warriors.

8

See the End Result and Be Nothing

"A mind unshaken by contact with the world. Sorrowless and stainless. Beyond the realms of suffering. The end of the obscuring defilements. Secure, once found it cannot be lost. This is a Blessing Supreme."
—Mangala Sutta—

It is not a matter of achieving, nor a matter of striving. It is a matter of simply being. This idea of striving suggests a gap, a gap where a union is necessary. "The ending is over there, and I am over here." This delusion of the gap must be dissolved into the pit of nothingness.

It will not be easy. After all, "I am here, my objective is over there. Countless obstacles are blocking my path. Once I clear these obstacles, I would have reached my destination." At least that is what the eyes see.

There would be, in essence, a conclusion to the story, a final chapter, if we may. Eat, sleep, and shit as the cow does. In other words, do not float away on a magic carpet with delusions of what time is. It exists for us all. If you are a mortal being reading these words, you entered this world and you will one day depart.

In Budo, there is an error in thinking that once you achieve the highest rank, you have attained all that is needed to know. You have earned your certificate, and you have graduated. This is also a reason many Budoka fall short and simply quit. Along the way, they will allow a poison of doubt to plant a seed. When times on the mat of the dojo floor get difficult, they may get bested in an arduous training session. They may lose a competition, get submitted, knocked unconscious, fail to get promoted or pass a test, or even suffer an injury.

These moments of temporary loss or disappointment hurt. They wound the soul, pierce your confidence. Then the seed of doubt grows into a weed, a weed that begins to extract life from the beginner's mind, which you once had. Then the untamed ego shows up, convincing you that this path you are on is not for you. Then, as if choking the final breath out of the last rose petal, the weed succeeds and you fall away. You quit.

In Zen, there is an outward appearance of inaction, yet a great presence of inward action. This action is to bring the mind home. This is the importance of Zen meditation: To not let the mind be invaded by poisonous seeds, to be awake in the now. As an active farmer, he regularly attends to his crops.

Every so often, a nail will uproot or stick out in the carpenter's floor. He has a choice: He can leave the nail sticking out, then others will be in danger of walking by and injuring their foot. Or he can remove it.

In the master carpenter's mind, every piece of wood has its use and every nail serves a purpose. His creation, from start to finish, began in his mind. He was, in essence, resolved from the beginning. His creation was already created from its birth, from its inception.

Incorrect measurements, faulty equipment, setbacks upon setbacks are all part of the process. When the carpenter sees things from this correct view, he will see that all setbacks and errors were not only for his learning but also for future generations.

Professor Renzo Gracie yelled, "Speech!" after he put the black belt around my waist. What I told all in attendance was that the black belt was not a destination, it was a glorious journey. So the correct view in Budo is not a large gem stone at the end of the trail. Instead, it is all the tiny gems, stones, and other small precious minerals that we can pick up along the way. When all is added up, there is indeed a glimmer that is gold.

I can recall a trip I made to Thailand. As we journeyed through the forest and up the mountain to see the great Buddha, the path was not easy. There were steep hills, and the Thailand forest seemed like a maze. The heat was well over a hundred degrees, so that made the hike even more difficult.

Being that Thailand was filled with stray dogs, it was not a strange thing to see a stray dog suddenly staring at you, even in the middle of a mountainous forest. As we approached what looked like a small, abandoned home, we realized that the house was protected by not one but at least 12 angry dogs, all of which suddenly emerged, barking at us viciously, showing their teeth, growling, and absolutely ready to attack. We had indeed trespassed; we were not welcome in their territory. Canines have an innate ability to smell fear. I was sure of three things: 1) I was going to finish this hike; 2) I would see the great Buddha at the top of the mountain; and 3) I was not going to die in Thailand getting eaten by hungry dogs.

Speed in a fight is critical. However, quickness of action is more important. Quickness of action goes beyond the speed of the physical body. In this case, we were terribly outnumbered.

Immediately I journeyed inward. I fortified my mind so that I was mentally ready to fight not one dog, but 100 dogs. I readied my spirit for a glorious battle to the end. I was resolved from the beginning. This mind-over-muscle eclipse instantly put me in a ready state instead of a fearful state.

Being this was near a small, rundown home of sorts, I moved slowly back and scanned the floor for an equalizing weapon. I knew any sudden movements would cause more aggression from the dogs, as they were getting more restless, barking louder, and foaming at the mouth. Near my right side lay a broomstick. A good weapon of choice; however, picking it up could prove fatal if done with the wrong energy.

My partner, who was in total fear, only added gasoline to the fire.

I had to find a way to be like water and put out the blaze. As I said before, an insight into a thing is compelling—it can give you sight beyond sight.

In Zen, there is something called function and form. What is the function of a broom? Simple, to sweep. When I simply made slow, sweeping actions toward the leaf and grass, the barking began to come to a halt. As I slowly retreated while sweeping, all aggressive attack dogs gradually became like curious puppies. Puzzled by the actions, they even became, for a moment, at peace.

Earlier that day, we had visited the Wat Chai Buddhist Temple. The head abbot asked me what our purpose was. I told him we were seeking a prayer, a spiritual blessing from the head monk for the mongkon, or headband that fighters wear before they engage in combat.

The head monk, a large man who had a piercing eye and was dressed in all white robes, arose, greeted us with prayer palms,

See the End Result and Be Nothing

then threw Thai holy water on the mongkon and us, all while wholeheartedly reciting the Thai sutras.

Then, with palms in prayer and his eyes closed, he returned the mongkon and simply said with a smile, "Go."

When we finally made it to the top of the mountain, along with the mongkon, to see the big Buddha, there was a wonderful sense of closure. However, that was not it.

I knew on that day that one day when I awoke, I would place the mongkon on the head of a worthy warrior. That warrior would do battle and be victorious. That warrior would simply see the mongkon as that, a headpiece of the Thai tradition, tightly woven threads, knotted together to make a beautiful headpiece of sorts—something that I asked them to wear.

On the contrary, it was all part of seeing the end result. There is no magic in the mongkon itself. Yet there is a Budo principle of sincerity that teaches you not to be attached to the material, but instead to be one with sincere action. So the key is to be nothing, yet see the totality of everything. If you are still trapped and see these words only as words, then you have not yet begun your journey.

The outer walk and all of its pain are necessary. It is a prerequisite to seeing the ego, for sometimes the ego is elusive. The best remedy is seeing, not seeing with the eyes. It is observing and hearing your two teachers.

The first teacher is the outer teacher. He may be a guru, master, or professor of some kind—a person whose very presence commands the utmost respect. This respect is a beautiful thing. It is the same respect you give to the sun or the moon for illuminating your path and providing you a way to go on your outward journey.

Then, there is the inner teacher. This teacher sits within all of us and is with us 24 hours a day, seven days a week. There is a particular interest to the inner teacher because he knows us well. We cannot put on a show for this teacher or hide our true feelings. He sees and knows all that we are. So the important thing is to remember that every good teacher was once a good student.

It is also important to keep with us each day a beginner's mind. Now, after the outward journey has begun, the merger of the outer and inner happen when we remain still and calm the mind. It is just as when you place a cup of cloudy water in a completely still position—both the outer and inner will merge. The cloudy will become unclouded, the cluttered will become uncluttered, the fixation of the one leaf will now see all leaves—you will dissolve into everything yet nothing, you will come upon that which is timeless.

This understanding is for those who intend to be warriors.

9

Go Through the Dark Side

*"Only a man who knows what it is like to be defeated
can reach down to the bottom of his soul
and come up with the extra ounce of power
it takes to win when the match is even."*
—Muhammad Ali—

Spit fire and chew nails. Chop sturdy wood, carry buckets of heavy water. I can only impart the concept of going through to the dark side. However, it is a personal journey that only you can take to understand fully. Also, there are a few teachings on this matter that I can impart only to students I train—those with a strong mind and people of the way.

The conditioning of the martial arts is a special thing. I have seen some of the most arrogant become the most humble simply through hard training. There simply is no short cut in terms of the conditioning that comes along with Budo training.

Journey Inward

Whether it is striking the makiwara hundreds of times, doing iron palm training for the hands, working many rounds on the heavy bag, or endless swings with the heavy suburito, the training is designed to make you do one thing: dig!

You must dig deep within yourself. You must journey inward. There you will see the core of yourself. It is a quiet place, a place that generally is not visited.

It is this place that can rest on the tip of a hair, yet it is so grand that it contains the totality of the universe. It is your spirit. What I have seen is that those who doubt the existence of spirit have not dug deep enough in the soil. The minerals and precious stones are deep. They are not on the surface. Many give up on the journey inward. They grow exhausted while digging and maybe even claim this is too difficult a task. Therefore, they do not make it down far enough. Those who are willing to remain steadfast, maintain discipline, and continue to dig will reach the grand horizon where the warriors dwell. It is a special place, reserved for the few.

During my time in Osaka, Japan, I was fortunate to visit Shitennoji Temple. As I sat inside the temple waiting for the monks to begin their service, I was expecting the usual liturgical chanting that is done in a Buddhist monastery. I am not a Buddhist but I can feel the Dharma in me and see it in the world.

One by one, the monks slowly filed in, tossing paper blessings and setting up positions to chant. Then, they began. It is difficult to convey in words what I heard that day. In essence, I felt as though I heard the sound of Budo. All the pain, all the blood, agony, sweat, tears, life, death, obligation, fears, laws, principles, masters, teachers, yin, yang, everything, and nothing.

The bass and acoustics of the temple had little to do with this. There were only about twelve or so monks, yet it sounded like

1,200. These particular sutras they were chanting date back many centuries. I could even envision warriors of that time reciting such sutra before going into battle or during a campaign at the death of a comrade. In other words, it was not only the sutra and its reverberating sound that resonated. It was where it was coming from.

It was coming from the gut, deep from within the belly of each monk. It is said that when chanting properly, you should say each word as if it were your last, as if you were connecting through your voice to the universe and all things around you. So, in essence, it is sung with the voice, but it is not a song. It is a matter of birth, life, death, and the wisdom of the ancients.

When I heard this, it was as if a fire had been lit in my soul. I knew then the importance of training the inner. And just as there are levels to the outer, white, blue, purple, brown, black belt, etc., there are also levels of internal training. Be that as it may, I still will say that spiritual practice is highly personal and what resonates with one may not resonate with another.

In music, we have keys or signature keys. Once a singer's voice is identified in a particular key, the musicians know what octave and pitch to play in. So in the key of G major, there will always be an F sharp. The F sharp is the signature key that will always be associated with G major.

If there is no knowledge of the key, the musician will have to use his ear to find the key. The signature key is the anchor, its principle, which pulls both voice and instrument together in harmony. So for me, Budo training was the anchor, the signature key. The sutra, once heard by my ear, was the key. It then became alive in a harmonious rhythm of wisdom—an inner, inner peace.

So why is it important to dig, to go so deep, when every ounce of your physical body tells you to stop, quit, go no more? Why must you push through? First, we must remember that we entered this world through a deep push from our mother's womb; there was a dig like no other to bring us into the world. So from the beginning, there was a beautiful struggle. We have an obligation to our parents to be thankful for their struggle, their push, their refusal to quit.

The Spartan–like conditioning of the martial arts comes out of the same spirit that birthed you into the world. The pain, the push, the constant demand that the teacher requires of you are all from the timeless, selfless motivation: love.

The conditioning necessary for a mixed martial arts bout is like no other on Earth, guaranteed. As a professional mixed martial artist, you must master the serpentine–like flow of Jiujitsu. You must know its 1,000 streets and avenues of entry points. You must guard those entry points. You must have a perfect plan to invade opponents' entry points. You must also have the limb dexterity to fight through an onslaught of submission holds. You must have the mental stamina inside a submission hold to defend not just the pressure of the submission hold, but also the potential strikes that can come along with that position. You must also have a thorough knowledge of throws—takedowns as well as takedown defense. You must have the strength to lift your opponent into the air and drive him to the canvas for takedowns. You must be able to enter correctly with proper footwork, to fit to the takedown of choice without getting hit along the way. You must have a body of steel and metal, as all bones will clash, shin to shin, knee to rib, elbow to skull, knuckle to mandible, and more. You must have the stamina to keep fast, sharp, accurate strikes of all kinds for at least twenty-five minutes, as a championship fight is five five-minute rounds. So the stamina must be superb at all levels and at every range. The breath is essential and the mind is important, yet the spirit is the most important.

As a police escort took us through the humid, drab streets of Sao Paolo, Brazil, it was interesting to see all the local people look at our traveling vehicle in awe. The locals all knew that a big event was going down that night. They knew that on that bus were today's top, modern-day gladiators. My student, Randy Brown, was set to fight against a game Brazilian fighter whose tokui waza was the guillotine choke. Due to his body type and aggressive style of fighting, he had a level of intensity that often led opponents to duck their head or expose their neck for this type of submission.

It is no secret that when I design training protocols for a fight, or gauntlets as they are often called, the training is absolutely brutal, to say the least. Most will not dare to take it. But those who can go to the side not illuminated by light, the dark side, which is within—those who can summon their best effort when it seems as nothing is there—will gain the advantage.

In one of our weekly gauntlets called spitfire, Randy had to push through rounds of full-contact, no rules–style sparring and do takedown rounds against the cage against elite takedown specialists. Then he had to do heavy positional and submission escape drills. After this, I demanded him to still have explosive power. He kicked the Thai pads, punched the heavy bags. Then he went through arduous conditioning for the core. In this drill, designed to protect the body, I slammed the dense Thai pad into his ribs and body at full force. This would happen repeatedly, nonstop. I was attempting to literally go through or strike through the fighter's body. If he did not breathe properly, he would collapse or fold under the intense impact.

Afterwards, we moved to a final drill, one that forces you to journey inward. Our grip strength is an interesting thing. Our grips go on a quick spike upward in strength, but sadly go in just as quick of a spiral downward once maximum grip strength is reached. In this drill, Randy would lock the rope with his best grip. I held his legs in the air. Then his task was simply to hold on, keep steady, and hang tight until the end of the timer.

As time progresses, the grip naturally becomes weaker. This is when the monsters come out, the dragons and demons that dwell in the underworld. These creatures of the underworld want you to give in, slip off, let go, give up. They are similar to those of the real world—haters who cannot wait to see you fail.

Our strength comes from a thorough knowledge of self and having the grit to bite down and keep pushing forward. This is an inward courage that manifests an outward vigor. As the entire team screams and shouts, supporting the fighter to go on, to hold on and to stay strong, all we have is our words and energy of support, which do help immensely. However, it is only you, who as my Sifu would say, can "go through that door."

On that day, function followed form, and Randy's mind and body were taxed. But they were still at one. He held on to the end, fingers on fire, writhing in fatigue, but he made it through to the other side. He had tamed the savage beast within.

As the chant, "*Uh via murrer*" ("You are going to die") roared through the stadium in Sao Paolo, what people did not know is that the way of the samurai is found in death. As the *Hagakure* states, "Even if a samurai's head is suddenly cut off in battle, he should still be able to complete one more action with certainty. When one becomes like a vengeful ghost and shows great determination, although his head is cut off . . . he will not die."

Randy's opponent was able to secure a choke called the mata leone (lion killer). Had he been able to apply full pressure, there would have been very little if no way to escape. However, only one thing stood between the full chokes closure and Randy's escape: Randy's grip.

In a fight, you will not rise to your level of expectation. You will fall to your level of training. Because Randy had gone through those doors of death countless times in practice, he was ready and prepared.

He has walked with me for quite some time down the path, and he is an elite exponent of warriorhood, fighting in the Ultimate Fighting Championship, the pinnacle of mixed martial arts competition.

As his opponent's depth to dig could not match Randy's depth to dig deeper, Randy escaped the submission and went on to defeat his opponent by submission. He was able to go through the dark side. The important thing is not to think of dark in terms of shades, tonation, or degrees of darkness as in the night. The correct view of this darkness we speak of is simple, yet few reach it. It is the unseen. It is that place within you that only you can reach. It is your personal abyss. It is a place you have to face yourself. You must absolutely rid your mind of any excuses, any nonsense of giving up or falling short of your own greatness. What then emerges is the light at the end of the tunnel. Here, it would also be wrong to understand this light as sunlight, a magical glow, or any such physical illumination.

What we should see it as is simple: that which is seen. Clarity and purpose. Again the metaphor of the flower emerges. It is not trying to look beautiful; it just is. For the martial artist, you will not try to act strong or try to be confident.

You are confidence, you are strength, you are rhythm, you are wisdom, you are experience, you are speed, you are courage, and you are victory. You have a mind like a spark, where there are no gaps, no hesitation. The concept of familiarization is understood. The spatial relationship is seen, the timing is mastered, you are inwardly steadfast and outwardly invincible.

It was a beautiful thing on that day to see the filled arena that cheered against us change from yelling, "Kill him" or "You are gonna die," to cheers of glory and praise within minutes. Every person applauded and gave a standing ovation. Randy dedicated that fight to his grandmother, who had passed away just a few days prior. In doing so, he gave life to her name forever. So on that day, his journey inwards also made all in attendance journey inward and find that when we discard outer trappings and attachments, what we are left with is only the truth. Void of any hometown favorites, void of a "my team vs. your team" mentality, void of all hindrances and duality, we come upon our true self, and this is a blessing supreme.

This understanding is for those who intend to be warriors.

10
Give Back

*"There are many kinds of postures in Karate,
while learning these postures should not be totally ignored, we
must be careful not to overlook that they are forms
or templates. It is the function of their application
that needs to be mastered."*
—Choki Motobu—

Sifu said, "Don't use tension. There will be a time for tension, but for now, you do not yet understand where to place the power. If you overexert yourself doing the form, you will merely burn out."

At that time, as a teenager I was so excited to be finally learning the highly sought out and secretive Art of Southern Mantis. In Kung Fu, there is a methodology for the use of power. The different styles provide different energy bases. Tiger claw may be more ferocious in approach, while crane may be more defensive and evasive. So when learning, it is critical to humble yourself and feel the master's hands. Much of what will be taught will be learned through feeling.

In order to learn this particular Art of Southern Mantis, my Sifu required first a certain level of loyalty. You could not just walk in and learn the Ph.D. science of Jook Lum Mantis. You first had to show a level of dedication to the Art and dedication to the school. At first, I did not understand his reasons. Later I would come to see exactly why this dedication is required.

First, there is the obvious. It is a credited course, just as in college. A certain number of credits are necessary before you register for a particular course. A certain amount of knowledge of body mechanics, conditioning, breathing, etc. is required. We needed to have a workman's knowledge of give and take, push–pull, and negative feedback.

Those were the fundamental reasons. But when we go deeper, we can see that Sifu was teaching us the lost art of appreciation. In today's world of martial arts, there is a fast-track approach. There are countless videos online or DVDs that you can purchase to begin to grasp the Art. You can have many questions answered, on your own time.

However, when you are learning under the eye of a watchful teacher, you will progress on his time. When he feels it is time and your level of understanding, sensitivity, and techniques is correct, there is a step-by-step approach. In this approach, a single answer, if given, is valued, treasured, like gold. Today's martial artists are spoiled. So many toys to play with and still they ask for more. I was fortunate to come up under a teacher who taught us how to build each working part of a single device. Thus, we appreciated the inner workings of that device and the device itself. The working parts were not given; they were earned. In mathematics, the teacher would often ask the student to show their work. In other words, do not simply say, "This plus this is that."

Show your work. How did you come to the total sum? If you use a calculator, you can just show the conclusion. It is not necessary to show the work. Our Sifu was helping us avoid becoming calculator Budoka—those who know only when told how to escape this, how to block that, etc. He was teaching us the spirit of the thing, which is ultimately to think for ourselves through the eyes of a martial artist.

The master teacher is not only watching your progression. He is quietly observing another, significant thing. That is, your ability to give back—to give back to the place where you learned and to help others who are starting out on their journey, such as helping the white belt who cannot tie his belt and assisting in teaching the mechanics to the beginners.

However, there is more, something ingenious in the traditional teachings, just as in Zen when a senior abbot will present a koan, which has no logical answer. It forces the Zen practitioner's mind to struggle. The mind naturally attempts to find a nearby solution. Then, what is realized is that time and experience reveal the answer. Experience and time are two critical aspects when teaching the martial arts. As a teacher, you realize that you are much more than a physical sports athletic coach. You are often a psychologist of sort, as students will come to you from all walks of life facing outside problems as well as problems on the mats.

By learning the traditional way of feeling the answer and finding clues, trial, and plenty of errors, your level of understanding is deeper. So your depth of helping others solve problems is more readily available, It is simple: You have gone down the path they are traveling many times before. You know the ins, outs, pitfalls, and pit stops. You can now begin to use wisdom to help guide them on their path.

The problems off the mat often affect the mind and spirit of the new trainee. Problems also depend on the student's age. They can range from being bullied at school, to divorce, depression, a suicide attempt, business bankruptcy, custody litigations, diagnosis of cancer, eviction, imprisonment, severe injury, loss of a relationship, loss of a loved one, loss of a job, and much more.

So you see, the martial arts are important, but martial living is more important. If I knew only how to punch and kick someone, I would be at a loss to help someone with deeper issues, such as a young man who is uncoordinated and shy but loves the martial arts, respects the dojo, and wants to learn; or a young girl who is handicapped, cannot use her arms as others can, and thus feels inadequate.

So you have a huge responsibility, not just to coach someone out of a depressed state from losing a match, but to observe them when they lose their match, to give them space, and to watch their ego. You are not only teaching the physical skills, but you must also learn to work with the ego and watch it carefully. The Budoka with a larger ego will often find excuses and hide, running away from their problem or going into denial. The Budoka with less of an ego will often be back on the mats the next day, with a relentless passion for seeing where they went wrong, understanding where they made an error, and asking how they can improve.

So as the great trainer Cus D'Amato taught, the coward and the hero feel the same in the face of danger, but it is what they do that makes them different. One walks toward the problem, while the other runs away.

So it is important to study, to read about the arts, to travel, speak with other martial artists, speak with other teachers, compare notes, analyze, revise and update, and constantly refine and polish the inner and the outer. Also study the teacher's teacher, someone called the grandmaster. Learn about their trials and errors, gain insight and inspiration. That which is happening now, has already been. There are not that many new things happening under the sun. Be sure to learn from the past masters. Some days you may need to call on their wisdom to give you guidance in helping another or yourself.

Satsujinken refers to the murderous sword or the sword that takes life. It can also, however, refer to destroying negative thoughts, emotions, and aspects of your character. Katsujinken is the life-giving sword. It would refer to overtaking an enemy without taking his life.

When we assist others on the path or begin teaching the martial ways, it is vital to understand these two concepts.

There was once a man who came into the dojo. He sat and watched class but asked to refrain from training in a group. He later explained that a close relative had been physically assaulted. Being that he had no fighting ability, he wanted to learn martial arts solely to seek revenge. He explained that he wanted to find the man and beat him to death. In essence, he wanted the murderous sword. I could fully understand his pain. There is a particular level of responsibility associated with wielding a sword. It must be put in the hands of a worthy warrior.

The fourth principle in our warrior code is compassion. Compassion is the principle that allows us to see through to the other side. In this case, I sympathized with his pain and let him know his anger was a righteous anger. But I told him that he should never put his passion before principle.

I also explained the degrees of karmic wind and how the type of people he is after often move in small degrees toward their own demise. One bad decision after another leads them to fall in the pit. Then, when the killer ghost of impermanence comes, their usual arrogance and forcefulness will run out. When we go chasing after such men of no account, we tie our karma to them. Sometimes we both fall in the pit, and sometimes we become the evil that we are chasing. The very thing we are trying to rid the world of is now in our soul. When this occurs, you lose.

Katsujinken, on the other hand, gives you the sky–like view, the ability to step back and see the sickness or attachments in our hearts and minds. According to what Yagyu Munenori said,

"Dust and dirt will become attached to rough, unpolished gems. The polished gem, however, will be flawless even in the midst of a swamp."

The class observer took my words to heart, and I am glad that he came to see me before acting on his own accord. He left the dojo in a heap of tears. He returned a few times simply to chat. Each time he looked better and better. He later joined our clan and learn the ways of the warrior.

Giving back is so much more than teaching someone to hurt; you also have to teach them how to heal. However, you cannot teach what is not instilled in you. Heijoshin, or true peace of mind, cannot be manufactured. When the teacher meets even the most beginner student, there is a path on which the teacher embarks to bring this student to the absolute best of their ability. On that path, one day the student surpasses the teacher, so the art can not only be preserved, it can improve.

So it is an important thing to know the seasoning of the master chef before you go adding your own spices. Walk closely to the master, ask questions, and truly listen to the answer. Then become those answers. Watch, look, listen, and observe.

When you teach, there is also learning. Suddenly an overwhelming sense of gratitude enters your heart when you try to teach others. You instantly realize it is quite difficult, especially depending on the attention span of whom you are teaching. My black belts who teach can attest to this. They then have almost a satori. It is so difficult to lead just one student to their ultimate potential. What about fifty or 100 students or more? Then there is a deeper understanding of the need for patience, compassion, and the sky–like view—especially for the uncoordinated beginner.

On some occasions, that beginner can remind you of someone very near: you. It is as if they are holding a mirror and you can see small areas of yourself. The student is sort of like a son, and the father can see himself in him. Yet just as the mirror does not get dirty or tarnished when it sees the flaws, so too must you remain untarnished, always taking the sky–like view.

It is there that you will begin to master your ego. Iron sharpens iron. The more you correct another, the more you reinforce the basics; the more you encourage a positive mind state, the more you bolster the enthusiastic beginner to harness his ability and you solidify your own.

When we give back, there is also a sense of purity. Good teachers expect nothing in return. They want only to see each student put forth their best efforts, be diligent in their practice, not slack off, and be the best possible version of themselves. Being able to defend himself and do well on the battlefield goes without question. However, a tide rises and falls, yet the ocean remains loyal and true.

This understanding is for those who intend to be warriors.

Instructions on Awakening

It is good to rise early, before the sun rises.

A good morning starts at night. Drink a nightly cleanse in a small amount. Apply liniments where needed. Apply minerals to the skin after daily practice. Fall and hit wine (dit dar jow) is best for calluses on the hands and shins.

Upon awakening, inhale first a breath of appreciation, then exhale a ready mind.

Make your bed.

Attend to yourself, then begin to prepare morning tea. Depending on the season, your combination may vary. Ginger and green tea are always good. Shilajit is as well; however, quality should be emphasized over quantity.

Prepare your zafu.

Journey Inward

Light one single incense. Do not neglect to clean your incense bowl; there should be fresh sand awaiting a single incense. Place the incense in the center.

Wear comfortable clothing. Attend to your animals; it is important to handle animals with care in the morning—they can see more than you are aware of.

Locate the text you wish to read, preferably an ancient text. Most writings of the ancients have fewer modern-day traps.

Stretch from head to toe. Start with the neck. Your spine is of great importance here. Then open the hips and stretch the hamstrings. Read while you stretch. Go into the deeper stretches; hold the stretch and read.

Sip your tea and begin breathing practice. I prefer Tai Chi, a meditation in motion. The sun will soon rise.

Now, sit as a sage on the zafu, eyes relaxed, legs folded, mind centered, aware of the breath.

Then, journey inward.

Gassho.

www.youtube.com/channel/UCLsWgbVvf5NmFLNe8JD6blg/

Closing

In closing, there are a few takeaway points that I want you to remember.

All healing, no matter what type, first starts within. The greatest doctor must study, the greatest artist must visualize, and the greatest musician must hear the rhythm within. First go within, connect the dots, strengthen within, then journey without.

The ego is not separate from you. It is not something to admonish. **You must go inward to find the ego and face yourself** through proper training, especially the methods I have set forward. You will make friends with your fears, you will be what Sun Tzu refers to as "a commander knowing troops." You are the commander; your thoughts and emotions fueled by the ego are your troops. You will take charge of orders given, you will take responsibility for actions made, and you will share both smiles and frowns of all campaigns.

With this mind, you will be at an advantage, for in situations of calamity, you will see opportunity. By learning to harness the trappings of the ego, you will keep your feet on the ground and be a genuine person. Others will feel your sincerity and see that you are a keeper of the way.

The last thing I will say is to remain steadfast, true, and

resolute. It will take courage to go within. Listen and adhere to the words of the masters. If your teacher is still living, go learn from them. **The important thing is hibi shoshin, which means to keep each day a beginner's mind.** Don't get attached to external confinements and traps. You must have an open mind and see learning as a gate. Take time each day to make the mind become new. Become a student of nature. Through stillness you will gain an insight into what hinders the mind. This will give you the ability to check the ego and remain at one with mind, body, and spirit, not losing your temper, not losing your center. As one of the elders said, "Profound peace, free of complexity, the natural simplicity. Beyond the mind of conceptual ideas, this is the depth of mind of the victorious ones."

About the Author

Sensei Nardu Debrah is a Senior full instructor in Universal Defense System under its Founder Sifu Ralph Mitchell, who is a Vietnam Veteran and Master Teacher of multiple Martial Arts. Sensei Nardu is also a 3rd Degree black belt in Brazilian Jiujitsu under the legendary Renzo Gracie, who is a Pride Fighting and UFC Veteran. Sensei Nardu is a professional mixed martial arts coach and former Ring of Combat champion. He has trained and developed Champions on all levels of Martial Arts Competition. He is the second born of Lisa Frazier. He started his journey in the Martial Arts at the age of 5 under his uncle Hassan Salahudin , a Veteran of the United States Marines and a student under the late Doctor Moses Powell. Sensei Nardu would later meet and train under the Vice President of the East Coast Kung Fu Federation Sifu Ralph Mitchell. Competing under Universal Defense System and team Renzo Gracie, Sensei Nardu went on to win multiple Chi Sao, Weapons, Full Contact Sparring events and Mixed Martial Arts Tournaments. He also holds victories in the World Eskrima Kali and Arnis Federation. Sensei Nardu is one of the early pioneers of MMA / No Holds Barred fighting in New York City. He has studied extensively the concepts of Jeet Kune Do under Sifu Ralph Mitchell. Trained in Muay

Thai, La Boxe Francaise Savate, Doce Pares, Kali/Arnis, fencing, Judo and Southern Mantis. He has had the opportunity to learn from his great Uncle Clarence Benyard of Bed–Stuy Boxing, the late George Washington and elder brother Kwabena Hardy. His MMA training has led him to meet and train under such experts as Rodrigo Gracie, Matt Serra, John Danaher and Yuri Silensky of Greco Roman Wrestling. As well as Robert Savoca Sensei of Brooklyn Aikikai and Kim Sensei of Toyama Ryu Batto do. His training has also led him abroad where he furthered his knowledge of Judo at the Kodokan in Japan as well as Iaido training in Kyoto. He also has trained Chen Style Tai Chi in China. He currently teaches Martial Arts at the Budokan Martial Arts Academy and exclusively for all who are serious to learn.

www.journeyinward.site

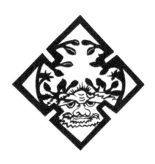

Glossary

Budo – A Japanese term. It means "martial way" and refers to those martial disciplines whose ultimate goal is spiritual, ethical, and/or moral self-improvement.

Budōka – A martial artist. Examples of Japanese Budo arts are Jiujitsu, Judo, Aikido, Karatedō, etc. The Sino-Japanese Kanji Bu means "military" or "martial"; The Kanji Dō has the semantics of the word "way." The suffix -*ka* corresponds to the Japanese character 家 with the meaning "family, house, home." Consequently, Budōka means "person who is or is at home in the martial arts of Budō."

Chiburi – Usually written 血振 in Japanese, literally means "shaking off blood." The image presented is that of flinging the blood of a defeated enemy off the blade with a sharp movement before resheathing.

Choji oil – A traditional Japanese blade-preserving compound. It is used in the maintenance of high-quality collectible blades. It contains clove oil extract and mineral oil.

Dit da jow – An analgesic liniment traditionally preferred by martial artists. Often a martial arts master blends his own mixture of aromatic herbs, such as myrrh and ginseng, which when combined are believed to stimulate circulation, reduce pain and swelling, and improve healing of injuries and wounds.

Doce pares – Spanish for twelve pairs or twelve equals, doce pares is a form of Arnis, Kali and Eskrima, or a Filipino martial art that focuses primarily on stick fighting, knife fighting, and hand-to-hand combat but also covers grappling and other weapons.

Escrima sticks – Used in the Filipino martial arts, Escrima sticks are the weapon of choice for many fans of the stick-fighting arts. In the Philippines, Escrima is a style similar to sword fighting and is sometimes referred to as Kali or Arnis de Mano.

Hasuji – The path your sword takes in a cut and the edge alignment whilst in that cut. A whistle as the sword whips through the air.

Hagakure – is a practical and spiritual guide for a warrior, drawn from a collection of commentaries by the clerk Yamamoto Tsunetomo,

Iaido – A Japanese martial art that emphasizes being aware and capable of quickly drawing the sword and responding to a sudden attack.

Jodan – Upper level, in this case referring to the level at which the sword is held.

Judo – A sport of unarmed combat derived from Jiujitsu and intended to train the body and mind. It involves using holds and leverage to unbalance the opponent.

Jujutsu – A method developed in Japan of defending oneself without the use of weapons by using the strength and weight of an adversary to disable him.

Kansetsu waza – Joint locks; consists of using one's own legs, arms, and knees, etc., to grasp the opponent's joint (elbow, knee, etc.) and bend it in the reverse direction to lock the joint.

Katsujinken – Life-giving sword.

Kawagane – The hard steel wrapping around the shingane. Shingane refers to the soft steel in the center of the blade.

Kokoro – Heart; mind; mentality; emotions; feelings in Chinese characters.

Makiwara – A padded striking post used as a training tool in various styles of traditional karate. It is thought to be uniquely Okinawan in origin.

Mekugi – (目釘) refers to a bamboo peg, which is inserted through mekugi-ana (目釘穴), so that the nakago(茎) is fixed to the sword hilt.

Mongkon – The mongkon is the headband worn by Muay Thai fighters before a fight. The headband itself is made by weaving together treasured material, such as the traditional Thai birth cloth, silk, and even hair from a loved one.

Mushin – The term is shortened from mushin no shin (無心の心), a Zen expression meaning, "the mind without mind" and is also referred to as the state of "no-mindness."

Nage-waza – A throwing technique; a Japanese term for a grappling technique that involves off-balancing or lifting an opponent and throwing them to the ground.

Ne-waza – Ground techniques; part of the katame-waza (grappling techniques) group. They include osae komi waza (hold-down techniques) and kansetsu waza (joint locks). As the name implies, these waza are performed on the ground and are used to hold an opponent down and disable his movement.

Noto – Resheathing the sword.

Reiho – A term that expresses the rules or abstraction of courtesy and respect, while "reigi" specifically means the techniques or actions of showing courtesy or respect.

Sankaku-jime – A triangle choke (三角絞), a type of figure-four chokehold that strangles the opponent by encircling the opponent's neck and one arm with the legs in a configuration similar to the shape of a triangle.

Satsujinken – Life-taking sword.

Saya – The Japanese term for a scabbard, specifically the scabbard for a sword or knife.

Sensei – Noun (plural same) (in martial arts) is a teacher. One who has gone before.

Shiai – (Judo and Karate) is a judo contest.

Shime-waza – A group of techniques that are all those involving constriction; strangulate.

Shinken (真剣, literally meaning "live sword") – A Japanese sword that has a live forged blade; the word is used in contrast with bokken and shinai. Shinken are often used for iaijutsu (combat practice) and/or tameshigiri (cutting) practice and/or Iaido.

Sifu – A title for and role of a skillful person or a master. The character 師/师 means "skilled person" or "teacher," while the meaning of 傅 is "tutor," and the meaning of 父 is "father."

Suburi – Repetitive individual cutting exercises used in Japanese martial arts such as Kendo, Aikido, Iaidō, and Kenjutsu. Often a shinai, bokken, suburitō, or even tanren bō are used.

Suburito – A type of bokken, a wooden practice sword. Heavier and thicker at the blade area.

Tai Chi – An internal Chinese martial art practiced for both its defense training, and its health benefits and meditation.

Tameshigiri – The practice of test cutting.

Tatami omote – A rush-covered straw mat forming a traditional Japanese floor covering. (*Omote* - Top layer.)

Uchiko powder – Made from finely ground whetstone. This is used to prevent rust and corrosion from developing on the sword blade.

Wat – A Buddhist monastery or temple.

Waza – The name for techniques performed in the seated stance in traditional Japanese (Koryū) martial arts. The word "waza" means "technique."

Zanshin – A state of awareness, of relaxed alertness, in Japanese martial arts. A literal translation of zanshin is "remaining mind." In several martial arts, zanshin refers more narrowly to the body's posture after a technique is executed.

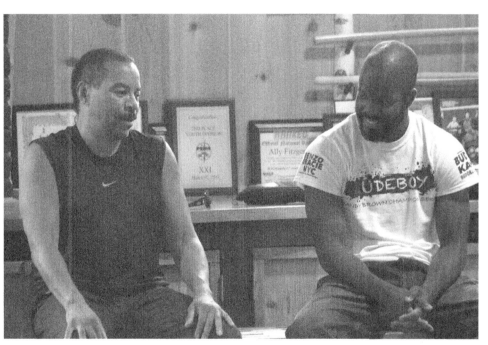
Precious gems from Sifu Ralph Mitchell

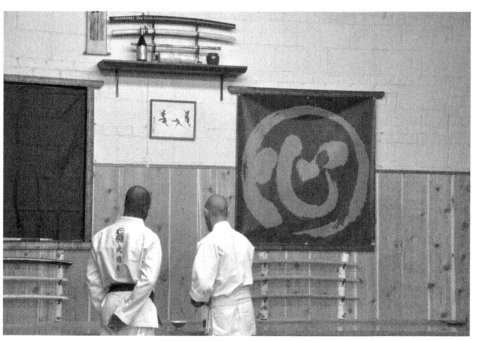

Lessons from Savoca Sensei

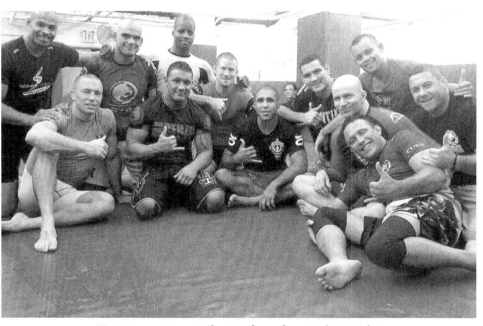

Training sessions at the Academy from Left to Right: David Branch, Bruno Tostes, George St.Pierre, Mark Cerrone, Myself, Josh Cholish, Gesias "JZ" Cavalcante, Chris Weidman, Magno Gama, John Danaher, Renzo Gracie and Jose "Zed" Chierghini

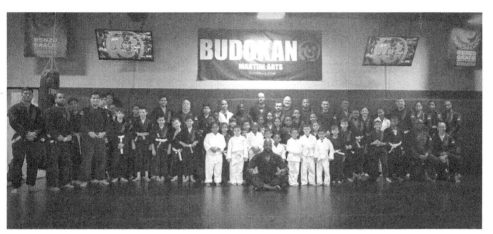

The wonderful students of the Budokan Martial Arts Academy

Made in the USA
Middletown, DE
08 April 2023

28465791R00066